An Examination of Emerging Bioethical Issues in Biomedical Research

PROCEEDINGS OF A WORKSHOP

Siobhan Addie, Meredith Hackma..., ...
Theresa Wizemann, and Sarah H. Beachy, *Rapporteurs*

Board on Health Sciences Policy

Health and Medicine Division

The National Academies of
SCIENCES · ENGINEERING · MEDICINE

THE NATIONAL ACADEMIES PRESS
Washington, DC
www.nap.edu

THE NATIONAL ACADEMIES PRESS   500 Fifth Street, NW   Washington, DC 20001

This activity was supported by a contract between the National Academy of Sciences and the National Institutes of Health (Contract No. HHSN263201800029I; Order No. 75N98019F00859). Any opinions, findings, conclusions, or recommendations expressed in this publication do not necessarily reflect the views of any organization or agency that provided support for the project.

International Standard Book Number-13: 978-0-309-67663-2
International Standard Book Number-10: 0-309-67663-0
Digital Object Identifier: https://doi.org/10.17226/25778

Additional copies of this publication are available from the National Academies Press, 500 Fifth Street, NW, Keck 360, Washington, DC 20001; (800) 624-6242 or (202) 334-3313; http://www.nap.edu.

Suggested citation: National Academies of Sciences, Engineering, and Medicine. 2020. *An examination of emerging bioethical issues in biomedical research: Proceedings of a workshop*. Washington, DC: The National Academies Press. https://doi.org/10.17226/25778.

The National Academies of
SCIENCES · ENGINEERING · MEDICINE

The **National Academy of Sciences** was established in 1863 by an Act of Congress, signed by President Lincoln, as a private, nongovernmental institution to advise the nation on issues related to science and technology. Members are elected by their peers for outstanding contributions to research. Dr. Marcia McNutt is president.

The **National Academy of Engineering** was established in 1964 under the charter of the National Academy of Sciences to bring the practices of engineering to advising the nation. Members are elected by their peers for extraordinary contributions to engineering. Dr. John L. Anderson is president.

The **National Academy of Medicine** (formerly the Institute of Medicine) was established in 1970 under the charter of the National Academy of Sciences to advise the nation on medical and health issues. Members are elected by their peers for distinguished contributions to medicine and health. Dr. Victor J. Dzau is president.

The three Academies work together as the **National Academies of Sciences, Engineering, and Medicine** to provide independent, objective analysis and advice to the nation and conduct other activities to solve complex problems and inform public policy decisions. The National Academies also encourage education and research, recognize outstanding contributions to knowledge, and increase public understanding in matters of science, engineering, and medicine.

Learn more about the National Academies of Sciences, Engineering, and Medicine at **www.nationalacademies.org**.

The National Academies of
SCIENCES · ENGINEERING · MEDICINE

Consensus Study Reports published by the National Academies of Sciences, Engineering, and Medicine document the evidence-based consensus on the study's statement of task by an authoring committee of experts. Reports typically include findings, conclusions, and recommendations based on information gathered by the committee and the committee's deliberations. Each report has been subjected to a rigorous and independent peer-review process, and it represents the position of the National Academies on the statement of task.

Proceedings published by the National Academies of Sciences, Engineering, and Medicine chronicle the presentations and discussions at a workshop, symposium, or other event convened by the National Academies. The statements and opinions contained in proceedings are those of the participants and are not endorsed by other participants, the planning committee, or the National Academies.

For information about other products and activities of the National Academies, please visit www.nationalacademies.org/about/whatwedo.

PLANNING COMMITTEE FOR A WORKSHOP ON AN EXAMINATION OF EMERGING BIOETHICAL ISSUES IN BIOMEDICAL RESEARCH[1]

JEFFREY KAHN (*Chair*), Andreas C. Dracopoulos Director; Core Faculty; Robert Henry Levi and Ryda Hecht Levi Professor of Bioethics and Public Policy, Berman Institute of Bioethics, Johns Hopkins University

ANITA LaFRANCE ALLEN, Vice Provost for Faculty, Henry R. Silverman Professor of Law and Professor of Philosophy, University of Pennsylvania

CECIL M. LEWIS, JR., Professor, University of Oklahoma

BERNARD LO, President, The Greenwall Foundation

MARIA MERRITT, Associate Professor, Berman Institute of Bioethics; Associate Chair, Student Matters, Department of International Health, Johns Hopkins University

CAMILLE NEBEKER, Associate Professor, University of California, San Diego, School of Medicine

BENJAMIN S. WILFOND, Director, Treuman Katz Center for Pediatric Bioethics, Seattle Children's Hospital and Research Institute; Professor and Chief, Division of Bioethics and Palliative Care; Department of Pediatrics; University of Washington School of Medicine

National Academy of Medicine Greenwall Fellow in Bioethics

RACHEL FABI, Assistant Professor, Center for Bioethics and Humanities, State University of New York Upstate Medical University

Board on Health Sciences Policy Staff

SARAH H. BEACHY, Senior Program Officer

SIOBHAN ADDIE, Program Officer

MEREDITH HACKMANN, Associate Program Officer

MICHAEL BERRIOS, Research Associate

KELLY CHOI, Senior Program Assistant

BRIDGET BOREL, Program Coordinator

ANDREW M. POPE, Senior Board Director

---

[1]The National Academies of Sciences, Engineering, and Medicine's planning committees are solely responsible for organizing the workshop, identifying topics, and choosing speakers. The responsibility for the published Proceedings of a Workshop rests with the workshop rapporteurs and the institution.

Reviewers

This Proceedings of a Workshop was reviewed in draft form by individuals chosen for their diverse perspectives and technical expertise. The purpose of this independent review is to provide candid and critical comments that will assist the National Academies of Sciences, Engineering, and Medicine in making each published proceedings as sound as possible and to ensure that it meets the institutional standards for quality, objectivity, evidence, and responsiveness to the charge. The review comments and draft manuscript remain confidential to protect the integrity of the process.

We thank the following individuals for their review of this proceedings:

MEGAN DOERR, Sage Bionetworks
MAYA SABATELLO, Columbia University
JULIE SCHUCK, The National Academies of Sciences, Engineering, and Medicine

Although the reviewers listed above provided many constructive comments and suggestions, they were not asked to endorse the content of the proceedings nor did they see the final draft before its release. The review of this proceedings was overseen by **DAN G. BLAZER II,** Duke University School of Medicine. He was responsible for making certain that an independent examination of this proceedings was carried out in accordance with standards of the National Academies and that all review comments were carefully considered. Responsibility for the final content rests entirely with the rapporteurs and the National Academies.

Contents

Boxes and Figure

BOXES

FIGURE

Acronyms and Abbreviations

ABPD   Association of Bioethics Program Directors
AI   artificial intelligence

CDC   Centers for Disease Control and Prevention
CHARM   Cancer Health Assessments Reaching Many
CPSC   Consumer Product Safety Commission

EHR   electronic health record
ELSI   ethical, legal, and social implications

FDA   U.S. Food and Drug Administration
FTC   Federal Trade Commission

HHMI   Howard Hughes Medical Institute
HHS   U.S. Department of Health and Human Services

IRB   institutional review board

LMIC   low- and middle-income country

NHGRI   National Human Genome Research Institute
NIH   National Institutes of Health

PAHO   Pan American Health Organization
PI   principal investigator

RCD   research, condition, and disease

STEM   science, technology, engineering, and mathematics

UC   University of California
UMBC   University of Maryland, Baltimore County

1

Introduction[1]

Biomedical research[2] has led to numerous discoveries and the translation of those advances into the areas of medicine, health, and policy for the purposes of improving health and reducing the burden of disease. Conducting responsible biomedical research and appropriately using and applying the new knowledge gained from these investigations in society will mean integrating the basic guiding principles of bioethics[3] into the translational process. Technological advances in biomedical research can lead to the appearance of new and emerging bioethical issues. The use of new technologies may also mean that existing bioethical challenges may be viewed in a new light. As scientific research, technological advances, and societal perspectives of those advances continue to evolve, ethical discussions are needed at the intersections where innovations meet the people who may

---

[1] This workshop was organized by an independent planning committee whose role was limited to identification of topics and speakers. This Proceedings of a Workshop was prepared by the rapporteurs as a factual summary of the presentations and discussion that took place at the workshop. Statements, recommendations, and opinions expressed are those of individual presenters and participants and are not endorsed or verified by the National Academies of Sciences, Engineering, and Medicine, and they should not be construed as reflecting any group consensus.

[2] "Biomedical research" refers to research that is broad in scope and can span disciplines of biology, medicine, behavioral, and social sciences. Conducting biomedical research may imply experimental inquiries to understand events at the atomic, molecular, cellular, organismal, and population levels (Flier and Loscalzo, 2017).

[3] "Bioethics" refers to the multidisciplinary study of, and response to, moral and ethical questions related to innovations in biomedicine (see What Is Bioethics at https://bioethics.jhu.edu/about/what-is-bioethics [accessed May 18, 2020]).

use them with the goal of ensuring that the benefits of research reach all individuals and that individuals are not subject to harms.

For example, as the use of digital technologies becomes ever more prevalent in daily life as well as in biomedical research and clinical care, new challenges related to informed consent, the privacy of patient information, responsible data sharing, and considerations for vulnerable and underserved populations are presented. Wearable technologies and applications on mobile devices passively collect biometric and behavioral data that can then be used for self-study or self-care, shared with health care providers, or used by the digital platform for purposes that the device owner might, or might not be, aware of. The potential ethical challenges can include issues related to health equity and health literacy (e.g., who has access to digital devices for participation in research) and a lack of data privacy protections for user-generated data that could be used to make conclusions about an individual's health. New models of biomedical research are emerging too, including patient-led research that takes place outside of the traditional regulatory environment (and often employs digital technologies). Individuals involved in citizen science[4] might fall into a less regulated area of research where the adherence to ethical research norms has less oversight. Another ethical challenge for the research enterprise in the United States is that certain populations have been consistently underrepresented in research (e.g., rural, low socioeconomic, and racial/ethnic minority groups), making it less likely that the benefits from research will be equitably distributed. Structural racism is a contributor to racial inequalities in health, and an examination of the origins of race can be helpful to begin to understand this important issue.

On February 26, 2020, the Board on Health Sciences Policy of the National Academies of Sciences, Engineering, and Medicine (the National Academies) hosted a 1-day public workshop[5] in Washington, DC, to examine current and emerging bioethical issues that might arise in the context of biomedical research and to consider research topics in bioethics that could benefit from further attention. The scope of bioethical issues in research is broad, and for this workshop the independent planning committee chose to focus on issues related to the development and use of digital technologies, artificial intelligence, and machine learning in research and clinical

---

[4]The term "citizen science" does not currently have a widely accepted definition, but has been referred to as "the general public engagement in scientific research activities when citizens actively contribute to science either with their intellectual effort or surrounding knowledge or with their tools and resources" (EC, 2014). Other terms for similar nontraditional research models include personal science, do-it-yourself science, patient-led research, or participant-led research. Citizen science is discussed in further detail in Chapter 3.

[5]The workshop agenda, speaker biographies, planning committee Statement of Task, and a list of attendees can be found in Appendixes A, B, C, and D, respectively.

practice; issues emerging as nontraditional approaches to health research become more widespread; the role of bioethics in addressing racial and structural inequalities in health; and enhancing the capacity and diversity of the bioethics workforce. Specific areas of research were outlined in the Statement of Task (see Box 1-1) as being out of scope for the workshop due to other ongoing projects in those spaces. The workshop was sponsored by the National Institutes of Health (NIH) Office of Science Policy.

CURRENT AND HISTORICAL SUPPORT
FOR BIOETHICS RESEARCH

Over the past 25 years many members of the bioethics community have benefited from funding from NIH, said Jeffrey Kahn, the director of the Johns Hopkins Berman Institute of Bioethics and the chair of the workshop planning committee. For example, support for bioethics from NIH has included bioethics-focused, investigator-initiated projects and research; inclusion of bioethics as a component in biomedical research projects; the embedding of bioethics researchers within biomedical research to examine and analyze the ethical issues raised; and support for trainees in bioethics-related programs.

Kahn said the majority of bioethics-related NIH research funding has been focused in three main areas: genomics, funded through the ethical, legal, and social implications (ELSI) portfolio that is administered by the National Human Genome Research Institute (NHGRI); the ethics of biomedical research, supported by several institutes of NIH; and bioethics capacity building outside the United States, through the funding portfolio administered by the Fogarty International Center. This support for bioethics research has been essential for the development of the field of bioethics and for the careers of many researchers, but Kahn said that it has also had the predictable effect of focusing bioethics research mostly into these three areas.

More recently, Kahn said, NIH has expanded its portfolio for bioethics research, including funding from the NIH Brain Research through Advancing Innovative Neurotechnologies (BRAIN) Initiative, which has explored neuroethics issues. Recent bioethics funding opportunities from NIH include administrative supplements[6] to support research on bioethical issues to inform policy development and funding from the National Center for

---

[6]See Notice of Special Interest: Administrative Supplement for Research on Bioethical Issues (Admin Supp Clinical Trial Optional), NOT-OD-20-038, https://grants.nih.gov/grants/guide/notice-files/NOT-OD-20-038.html (accessed April 29, 2020); and Notice of Special Interest: Administrative Supplements for Research on Ethical, Legal and Social Issues regarding Post-mortem Pediatric Tissue Procurement for Research Purposes (Admin Supp Clinical Trial Optional), NOT-OD- NOT-HD-20-012, https://grants.nih.gov/grants/guide/notice-files/NOT-HD-20-012.html (accessed April 29, 2020).

BOX 1-1
Workshop Statement of Task

A planning committee of the National Academies of Sciences, Engineering, and Medicine will be appointed to conduct a 1-day workshop to bring together stakeholders to discuss potential ethical issues that may arise from new and emerging trends in biomedical research (including behavioral and social research) and society. The workshop will identify a range of current and emerging bioethical issues—both in basic and clinical research—and explore a broad range of stakeholder perspectives. Input will be sought from a variety of perspectives which may include patients/participants/individuals, bioethicists, academic and industry researchers, clinicians, and government representatives. The workshop will describe the state of the emerging science and potential pressing, recurring, emerging, and/or anticipated future bioethical issues in biomedical research and society that fall within the scope of the research and policy activities of the National Institutes of Health. Potential topics may include

- Use of digital technologies, artificial intelligence, and machine learning in biomedical research and clinical care;
- Emerging ethical challenges for sharing data from human research participants and use of human biospecimens;
- Health equity and health disparities in research, including
  o Recognizing and addressing barriers to participation in research and clinical care across diverse populations and groups,
  o Understanding the impact of cultural and social context on health and disease, and
  o Equitable distribution of the benefits and burdens of research;
- Innovative study designs, including crowdsourcing of research and citizen science;
- Novel approaches for enhancing bioethics infrastructure and training;
- New means for assessing and enhancing scientific workforce diversity; and/or
- Innovative solutions for enhancing research oversight infrastructure.

Given the broad scope of bioethical issues in research and the difficulty in addressing all possible issues in a single workshop, the following topics fall outside the scope of this workshop as they are being addressed in multiple other venues: gene editing, gene drives, human–animal chimera research, human fetal tissue research, neuroethics, and animal care and welfare. The planning committee will develop the agenda for the workshop, select and invite speakers and discussants, and moderate or identify moderators for the discussions. Workshop proceedings will be prepared by a designated rapporteur based on the information gathered and discussions held during the workshop in accordance with National Academies institutional policies and procedures.

Advancing Translational Sciences[7] to support the study of ethical issues in translational science research.

Although the NIH bioethics portfolio continues to expand, it is still limiting researchers in some ways, Kahn said, as there are many bioethics topics, and approaches to studying them that do not fall within the current NIH funding portfolio. This workshop is an important beginning to the discussion of how that research portfolio might be expanded further and create new opportunities, Kahn said (see Box 1-1).

It is important to note that the World Health Organization declared COVID-19 a pandemic on March 11, 2020, 2 weeks following this workshop. At the time of the workshop, there was limited evidence of community spread in several U.S. states, and widespread physical distancing efforts had not yet been implemented in the United States. As such, speaker remarks were focused broadly on bioethical issues in biomedical research and clinical care that were not related specifically to COVID-19. On March 27, 2020, the Coronavirus Aid, Relief, and Economic Security (CARES) Act was signed into law, expanding reimbursement for telehealth and remote patient monitoring under Medicare.[8] Other large private payers, including Aetna, Cigna, and Blue Cross Blue Shield, have also expanded coverage of telehealth in their health plans.[9] The Office for Civil Rights at the U.S. Department of Health and Human Services (HHS) issued a statement in mid-March 2020 indicating that it would be exercising enforcement discretion about the Health Insurance Portability and Accountability Act of 1996 rules regarding remote communications technologies used for telehealth during the pandemic.[10] Given this rapidly evolving landscape, there may be additional bioethical issues related to digital technologies, structural racism and health disparities, privacy, and other topics that were not expressly covered during the workshop and that warrant further discussion as well as additional funding opportunities. For example, at the time of publication,

---

[7]See Ethical Issues in Translational Science Research (R01 Clinical Trial Optional), RFA-TR-20-001, https://grants.nih.gov/grants/guide/rfa-files/RFA-TR-20-001.html (accessed April 29, 2020).

[8]For more information about the CARES Act, see https://www.congress.gov/bill/116th-congress/house-bill/748 (accessed April 27, 2020).

[9]For more information on private payer coverage of telehealth, see https://www.aetna.com/individuals-families/member-rights-resources/covid19/telemedicine.html, https://www.cigna.com/coronavirus, and https://www.bcbs.com/coronavirus-updates (all accessed April 27, 2020).

[10]For more information on HHS enforcement discretion related to telehealth remote communications, see https://www.hhs.gov/hipaa/for-professionals/special-topics/emergency-preparedness/notification-enforcement-discretion-telehealth/index.html (accessed April 27, 2020).

NHGRI had issued a new funding opportunity for ELSI research related to COVID-19.[11]

OVERVIEW OF TOPICS HIGHLIGHTED DURING PRESENTATIONS AND DISCUSSIONS

A number of topics were discussed throughout the workshop sessions as participants considered the range of bioethical issues that are relevant to biomedical research. While the workshop was funded by NIH, the meeting day aimed to cover material that would be of value to many groups in the fields of bioethics and biomedicine, including academic researchers and funders from the United States and around the world. While several of the presenters provide considerations for NIH, the issues raised during the discussions may also be of interest to other stakeholders. The topics highlighted below were drawn from individual speakers' remarks and the open discussions and are addressed further in the succeeding chapters.

Ethical Norms

Several times during the workshop speakers acknowledged that data scientists and digital technology developers currently operate under a very different set of cultural norms, ethical commitments, and incentive structures than those of biomedical research and health care practice. Some speakers said that a better understanding of ethical issues is needed by digital technology developers and data scientists but that those efforts will also need to be supplemented by guidelines, regulations, system architecture, collaboration among various stakeholders, and improved incentive structures.

Multidisciplinary Collaboration

Collaboration among biomedical subject-matter experts and algorithm developers was discussed as being essential for the development and assessment of safe, reliable, and useful tools for health. Importantly there was also discussion about the potential value of designing bioethics research projects that draw from multiple disciplines, including law, philosophy, sociology, history of medicine, critical medical humanities, science and technology studies, and literary theory. Some speakers felt that it would be advantageous to pair bioethics research questions directly with scientific innovation.

---

[11]See Notice of Special Interest regarding the Availability of Urgent Competitive Revisions for Research on the 2019 Novel Coronavirus, NOT-HG-20-030, https://grants.nih.gov/grants/guide/notice-files/NOT-HG-20-030.html (accessed April 29, 2020).

Workforce Training

Training was a recurrent theme across panel discussions in terms of incorporating bioethical principles into various biomedical fields and for the purposes of preparing the bioethics workforce itself. As an example of integrating bioethics into other fields, it was discussed that the field of data science is in the early stages of addressing key ethical issues but that attention is now being paid to ethics challenges. It was mentioned that scientific conferences are devoting sessions or entire meetings to ethical issues and that colleges and universities are implementing ethics classes for data scientists. Speakers also shared their thoughts on the need for training clinicians and clinical laboratory professionals in the proper and unbiased use of algorithms. With regard to developing the bioethics workforce, it was discussed that bioethics training is reaching people too late in their careers and that there is a need to attract a more diverse group of people to the field of bioethics at an earlier age, including supporting doctoral research in bioethics. There was also discussion of the limitations of current bioethics training programs for research professionals. The importance of taking country context into account in training programs for bioethicists was also noted by speakers at the workshop as well as the value of training ethicists for transdisciplinary research.

Transparency and Choice in Data Sharing

There was much discussion about individuals' awareness of, understanding of, and ability to consent to the sharing and uses of their health and medical data. Participants discussed the value of transparency and choice when individuals must agree to the sharing of their data in order to receive services and when shared data are not subject to appropriate governance. Participants also discussed the differences between data sharing within the context of a research collaboration (where responsibilities and ethical norms are preserved) and the sale or transfer of data (where control is often relinquished).

Racism and Structural Inequalities

The impact of racism and structural inequalities was discussed relative to issues such as the development of digital technologies and disparities that can be introduced by their use, who participates in research and why they do or do not, and who has the opportunities to be trained for careers in the biomedical and bioethics fields. For example, it was discussed that biases in the data used to train machine learning algorithms can result in structural inequalities that perpetuate inequalities. Participants also discussed some of the historical context and current reasons why underrepresented populations often do not participate in research.

Power and Privilege

Implicit biases and structural forces assign status to people, which in turn may create differences in power and privilege. The concept of power and privilege was discussed in the context of the conduct of research—specifically, who has the right to formulate the questions, to define benefits and harms, and to define what qualifies as "success." Workshop participants observed that professional researchers, who traditionally hold the power, often have not had the same lived experience as people from minority communities or individuals conducting self-study and often make the mistake of assuming they know what is needed by the people they are working to serve.

Research Questions for Funding or Focus

One of the objectives of the workshop was to consider potential research topics in the areas of bioethics as it relates to the use of digital technologies, data collection and use, citizen science, structural inequalities around who participates in research, and the workforce training infrastructure for bioethicists. A broad range of ideas were suggested by individual participants throughout the workshop for further attention and funding support, and these ideas are included in Chapter 6.

ORGANIZATION OF THE WORKSHOP AND PROCEEDINGS

This Proceedings of a Workshop summarizes the presentations and discussions that took place at the workshop on February 26, 2020. The first two panel sessions focused on the ethical issues associated with the use of digital health technologies, artificial intelligence, and machine learning in biomedical research and clinical care (Chapter 2). The third panel considered the different forms of innovative research models that are participant-led or patient-centered (compared with scientific investigator–led), such as citizen science, that take place outside of the traditional regulatory environment. Panelists discussed other forms of citizen science, such as personal science, and the governance of unregulated research involving mobile devices and how people pursuing these types of studies might do so ethically (Chapter 3). The next panel examined the impact of inequality on health, disease, and who participates in research. Panelists discussed race, racism, structural inequalities, the lasting impacts of historical ethical failures and harms, and the unique issues affecting sovereign tribal nations (Chapter 4).

This was followed by a discussion of bioethics workforce issues, including training needs and opportunities to ensure and maintain diversity in the workforce (Chapter 5). The workshop concluded with observations and reflections shared by panelists from a variety of agencies that fund bioethics research and from audience participants (Chapter 6).

2

Ethically Leveraging
Digital Technology for Health

Highlights of Key Points Made by Individual Speakers

- Digital technologies are being increasingly used in self-care, clinical care, and biomedical research, and it is important that developers consider ethical components in the design process. Potential risks such as exposure of private information will likely need to be addressed by both law and better system architecture. (Estrin)
- There is a wide range of potential ethical risks associated with the use of digital technologies, including privacy exposure and re-identification of anonymized data; the use of one's data for purposes beyond the original intent without one's knowledge or consent, including selling to commercial entities; the discriminatory use of shared data; the collection and use of poor quality data; and inadvertent inclusion in research by association. (Mello)
- Many of the ethical concerns associated with emerging digital technologies cannot be adequately addressed within the existing regulatory system and should take into account different views on data privacy and intergenerational shifts in privacy perceptions. (Mello)
- Research is needed to explore how research participant literacy can be improved so that participants have a better understand-

ing of how research is conducted; how data are collected, stored, and shared; and how a technology works (Nebeker, Ossorio)

- Machine learning algorithms can be inherently biased as a result of inadequate data, asking bad questions, a lack of robustness to dataset shift, dataset shift due to evolving health care practice, model blind spots, and human errors in design. Metrics and tests should be developed to measure whether an algorithm is biased. (Saria)
- Safe and reliable machine learning in health care involves understanding how artificial intelligence tools work, being able to determine if they are working, and ensuring they continue to work as expected. (Saria)
- Collaboration among subject-matter experts and algorithm developers is essential for the development and assessment of safe, reliable, useful tools, and standards are needed to help ensure responsible implementation in health care practice. (Ossorio)
- Data scientists and digital technology developers operate under a very different set of cultural norms, ethical commitments, and incentive structures than those of biomedical research and health care practice. (Estrin, Mello, Ossorio)
- Machine learning algorithms for use in health care should be held to rigorous standards, similar to those for the development of drugs. (Ossorio, Saria)

The use of digital health technologies, artificial intelligence (AI), and machine learning in biomedical research and clinical care was discussed during the first two panel sessions. A range of ethical concerns can emerge in the development and implementation of new science and technologies, said Bernard Lo of The Greenwall Foundation and moderator of the sessions. Deborah Estrin, an associate dean and the Robert V. Tishman '37 Professor at Cornell NYC Tech, provided an overview of the digital health technology landscape, and Michelle Mello, a professor of law and medicine at Stanford University, discussed ethical issues associated with emerging digital health technologies. Suchi Saria, the John C. Malone Assistant Professor in the Department of Computer Science and the Department of Health Policy and Management at Johns Hopkins University, reviewed the state of AI and machine learning in biomedical research, and Pilar Ossorio, a professor of law and bioethics at the University of Wisconsin, discussed ethical issues associated with the use of machine learning, including deep learning neural networks, in health care.

DEVELOPING, TESTING, AND INTEGRATING DIGITAL TECHNOLOGIES INTO RESEARCH AND CLINICAL CARE

Overview of the Digital Health Technology Landscape

Estrin said current and emerging digital technologies are increasingly being used in self-care, clinical care, and biomedical research across four main categories: wearables, mobile applications (apps), conversational agents, and digital biomarkers. Moreover, technologies such as mobile phones have been used to support care delivery for more than a decade (e.g., by community health workers in resource-limited settings).

Wearables for Biometrics and Behavior

Wearables are mobile devices that measure and track biometric data such as heart rate, activity, temperature, or stages of sleep, Estrin said. Some examples of wearables include activity and sleep trackers and smart watches by Fitbit, Garmin, Apple, and Oura, to name a few. She noted that the availability and usability of wearables have increased dramatically since the early days of actigraphy (noninvasive monitoring of cycles of movement and rest). Even if current wearables do not meet clinical standards, she said, they can track trends; most wearables are used in association with a companion mobile app that provides the wearer access to data summaries.

The increasing ability of machine learning algorithms to interpret the data collected by wearables is enhancing the utility of those data for individuals in self-care decision making as well as for use in guiding clinical care and informing research. For example, Estrin suggested, a wearable might help an individual better understand how exercise, diet, and alcohol consumption contribute to his or her poor sleep patterns; the clinician might use the data to evaluate the effectiveness of interventions to reduce the impacts of poor sleep quality on cognition or metabolism; and the data can help inform research on interventions to improve sleep quality.

Mobile Apps

There are also stand-alone mobile apps that are used independently of a wearable digital device. These mobile apps are focused on an interaction with the patient for self-care, for clinical engagement (e.g., to encourage adherence to a treatment plan), or for research purposes. Estrin briefly described four categories:

- Symptom Trackers—This category of mobile app allows individuals to enter symptoms and see how they change over time. One example, Estrin said, is the Memorial Sloan Kettering Cancer Center symptom tracker. Using the mobile app, patients recovering from surgery and undergoing treatment can track their symptoms and plot their data against expected results. This interactive approach allows patients to see their progress and better evaluate if they are progressing sufficiently to avoid an unnecessary emergency room visit.
- Access to Clinical Health Records—Mobile apps are also used to provide individuals with access to their clinical health records. Estrin said that Apple HealthKit and Android CommonHealth are developer platforms that take advantage of data interoperability standards, such as Fast Healthcare Interoperability Resources, to provide access to electronic health records (EHRs). App developers can use these platforms to create apps that allow users to access and share their clinical health information securely.
- Health Behavior Apps—Another category is health behavior apps that provide coaching and guidance for individuals on choosing healthy behaviors. Examples include diabetes prevention programs such as Omada, the Noom app for weight loss, and the Livongo apps, which support health goals across several conditions. Some health behavior apps have been shown to have a positive effect on behavior, Estrin said, but many others have not been vetted or tested.
- Behavioral Health Apps—The final category, which involves behavioral health, is different from health behavior apps because of the focus on mental health support, Estrin said. PTSD Coach, developed by the U.S. Department of Veterans Affairs, was an early example of a behavioral health app, which provides "in-the-moment support" based on clinical guidelines. Other examples of behavioral health apps include Talkspace, LARK, and HealthRhythms.

Conversational Agents

Conversational agents are chatbots and voice agents, many of which can be accessed via digital assistants such as Google Home and Alexa, are programmed to hold a conversation in a manner similar to a human. Examples of emerging health-specific conversational agents include Sugarpod for diabetes, Kids MD by Boston Children's Hospital, and other chatbots for use by patients, nurses, and home health aides. Some conversational agents are entirely automated, and others provide details to a human provider or coach, Estrin said, but starting with an automated interaction to address more routine concerns allows providers to better meet and manage client needs.

Digital Biomarkers

Digital traces (i.e., records of online activity) are also being explored as digital biomarkers, Estrin said. For example, she said, researchers have collected data for mood analysis from social media interactions[1] and others have used individual Internet search data as indicators of health status.[2] Another example is an institutional review board (IRB)-approved retrospective study by Northwell Health of the Internet searches done by individuals prior to their first hospital admission for a psychotic episode.[3] Individuals in the study consented to sharing their Google search history (via Google's Takeout data download service), which is used by researchers to look for temporal patterns of online searching, location data, and other online activity that are associated with serious mental illness. Such research seeks to inform specific models for how to use such data to inform care at a population and individual level.

Risks and Concerns Related to Digital Technologies

Potential ethical risks and concerns associated with the use of digital technologies in research and clinical care include privacy exposure when using these digital technologies for health-related surveillance, data use, and transparency around AI-assisted agents, Estrin said. How the data should be controlled depends on the context of use, Estrin explained, and she said that laws and system architectures addressing how data are shared for surveillance need to take the context of use into account. Contextual integrity allows for a more nuanced view of privacy issues than traditional dichotomies (Nissenbaum, 2018). It exposes the risks associated with how an individual's data flow and how they are used. The use of unquestioned consumer-app terms of service for health-related apps might allow the app provider to sell a user's health data. There are some concerns that health data should be protected differently in order to prevent its use in discriminatory ways related to insurance coverage, employment, issuing credit, or dating, for example. This may require legal, as well as technical, protections, Estrin said. Another concern is transparency with regard to when an individual using a digital health technology is interacting with an AI agent (i.e., a "softbot" or software robot) or a human agent. A question for consideration is whether or when it is the right of patients to know if they are interacting with a person or an AI-mediated agent, she said.

---

[1]For more information, see Saha et al., 2017.
[2]For more information, see White et al., 2018.
[3]For more information, see Kirschenbaum et al., 2019.

ETHICAL ISSUES FOR EMERGING DIGITAL TECHNOLOGIES

The increasing use of individuals' data traces in novel ways for both research and clinical care challenges the norms of human subjects research ethics and existing privacy laws, Mello said. Existing research ethics concerns have been heightened by the advent of new digital technologies, she said, and new concerns have also emerged as the use of digital technologies has expanded (summarized in Box 2-1).

Existing Concerns Compounded by Digital Technologies

Purpose and Repurpose

Existing concerns about purpose and repurpose center on the informed consent process and the extent to which data and biospecimens generated for one purpose may be used for other purposes without securing fresh consent. These concerns now encompass data generated by digital technologies, including whether such data can be shared or sold for research purposes. The digital data of interest for research might include data from user interactions with apps and websites and clinical data generated by digital technologies in the care setting (e.g., ambient listening devices such as surgical black boxes).[4] Data mining raises additional concerns since the research is often not hypothesis-driven but exploratory. It is also possible that unrelated datasets might be linked for research or clinical purposes. As highlighted by a legal complaint filed by a patient in 2019 against Google and The University of Chicago, EHR data collected for clinical purposes may be transferred to private companies for the purpose of developing new commercial products,[5] and even with direct identifiers removed they are potentially re-identifiable through linkages to other data (e.g., linking smartphone geolocation data to the EHR data could reveal which clinics a patient has visited, when, and for what purpose) (Cohen and Mello, 2019). Once a patient is re-identified, Mello said, the EHR data could potentially be linked to other data such as social media and online browsing activity.

The three main solutions that have generally been used to address concerns about purpose and repurpose have been de-identification, waiver of consent, and blanket consent, Mello said, adding that there are issues with each approach. De-identification is "infinitely harder" for digital data than for tissue specimens. Consent waivers, granted when an IRB determines

---

[4]Surgical black boxes can record a range of data during surgical procedures, including videos of the procedure, conversations in the room, and ambient conditions for the purpose of identifying intraoperative errors that may have led to adverse events.

[5]For more information on *Dinerstein v. Google*, see https://edelson.com/wp-content/uploads/2016/05/Dinerstein-Google-DKT-001-Complaint.pdf (accessed April 20, 2020).

BOX 2-1
Existing and Emerging Bioethical Concerns
Associated with Digital Health Technologies

Existing Concerns Compounded by Digital Technologies
- **Purpose and repurpose**—Data and biospecimens generated for one purpose may be used for other purposes without securing fresh consent.
- **Context transgressions**—Expectations of privacy vary depending on the context, yet data uses may transcend originally envisioned contexts (Nissenbaum, 2011).
- **Corporate involvement**—Digital technology companies are not governed by the traditional structures for ethical oversight in biomedical research.
- **Incidental research subjects**—Individuals can inadvertently come under the observation of researchers simply by their incidental association with others who are sharing data.

Emerging Issues
- **The scale of data collection**—Vast amounts of data can now be collected with minimal cost and effort, and concerns include data privacy, data quality, and social consequences (e.g., stigmatization, discrimination).
- **The end of anonymity**—The re-identification of individuals using data from putatively de-identified datasets is now increasingly possible due to advances in computer science.
- **The ethical adolescence of data science**—Although training and acculturation in science and medicine convey a strong, clear set of ethical norms and sense of professionalism, this is not yet the case for computer scientists, yet digital technology companies enjoy a high degree of autonomy, with few external ethical controls.

SOURCE: Michelle Mello workshop presentation, February 26, 2020.

---

that the research meets certain requirements and therefore some or all consent elements can be waived, are a practical solution in the sense that securing fresh consent is often impracticable, Mello said, but they are not a principled solution to the problem of informed consent for repurposed digital information.[6] Blanket consent might be a more transparent solution, she continued, but it arguably is not meaningful consent if researchers

---

[6]A waiver of informed consent (45 CFR 46.116) can be granted by an IRB if research involves minimal risk to participants, if research cannot be conducted practically without a waiver, if the waiver does not negatively affect the rights of the participant, and if participants will be provided additional information about their participation following the study (when applicable). Blanket consent refers to a research participant consenting to all uses of their data with no restrictions.

cannot explain to participants the potential range of uses of their data and the potential for future data linkages. The field needs to think deliberately about the issue of informed consent for repurposed digital information, Mello said, and there may be real limits to using transparency as a strategy given the challenges with adequately describing what participants are consenting to and the lack of choice that many users of digital technologies have about accepting the terms of use.

Context Transgressions

Individual expectations of privacy vary depending on the context, Mello said, reiterating the point made by Estrin. Expectations are influenced by the relationship one has with whomever is receiving one's information and by how one expects that information to be used (Nissenbaum, 2011; Sharon, 2016; Solove, 2020). Furthermore, she said, empirical research has found that the willingness to provide one's information varies significantly depending on whether that information is expected to be used for noncommercial or commercial purposes. For example, how a person feels when one of that person's doctors shares very sensitive clinical information with other health care providers (e.g., to coordinate care) can be very different from how that person feels about social media platforms (e.g., Facebook) sharing much less sensitive information about him or her with other entities for commercial purposes.

The problem of transgressions of context is related to the problem of purpose and repurpose, but it is distinct, Mello said. Historical examples of context transgressions include the case of Henrietta Lacks[7] and the case of *Moore v. Regents of University of California*,[8] both of which involved an individual's property rights, or lack thereof, in relation to commercial products derived from the person's biospecimens.[9] For rapidly exchanged digital information, the potential for transgressions of context is very high, Mello said—in particular, via the shift in context from noncommercial to commercial uses of data. A current example is health care organizations transferring large volumes of EHR data to technology companies for use in developing commercial products and services.

Addressing potential context transgressions has generally involved clearly disclosing that individuals do not have any rights to a share of the

---

[7]For more information, see https://www.hopkinsmedicine.org/henriettalacks/upholding-the-highest-bioethical-standards.html (accessed April 20, 2020).

[8]For more information, see https://law.justia.com/cases/california/supreme-court/3d/51/120.html (accessed April 20, 2020).

[9]In each case, cancer cells collected from patients Henrietta Lacks and John Moore in the course of their clinical care were used to develop cell lines that were later commercialized, without the patients' knowledge or consent.

profits from technologies developed from their biospecimens, Mello said, or removing any information identifying the individual, or both. Alternatively, commercial and noncommercial context transgressions could be avoided by simply not sharing information, but Mello said this strategy is neither feasible nor desirable because needed products and services stem from data sharing. Another approach could be to eliminate the expectation of privacy altogether and make individuals aware that they are relinquishing control of their information in exchange for a variety of current and future benefits (e.g., free and low-cost services, development of precision medicine technologies). This approach conflicts with current privacy laws and human subjects protections, she said, and would shift the data sharing model from one of individual control over data to one of group deliberation and benefit sharing.

Corporate Involvement

For-profit corporations, including pharmaceutical companies and others, have long been involved in biomedical research, Mello said, and concern about the influence that corporations have on research persists. Digital technology companies have now emerged as dominant forces in biomedical product development. When they are not partnering with academic researchers or government, digital technology companies operate outside the ambit of structures that traditionally have provided ethical oversight of biomedical research (e.g., IRBs), Mello said, and comparable ethics mechanisms are largely absent in the industrial sector. Furthermore, digital technology companies have developed sufficient analytic capacity that they no longer need to interact with academic biomedical researchers for anything except to acquire patient data. The need for that interaction is also declining since digital product developers can often obtain health information directly from consumers or from direct-to-consumer companies. Corporate involvement is essential for product development, she said, but there are many issues yet to be addressed.

Incidental Research Subjects

Incidental research subjects are individuals who have not consented to be research participants but who have inadvertently come under the observation of researchers by association with others who are sharing data. Incidental sharing of information is a concern in the field of genetics, for example, where one person's genomic data can reveal information about family members. The digital version of the problem is much broader, Mello said. For example, digital technologies such as ambient listening devices collect all conversations, not just those of the device owner, and digital traces such as social media posts can sweep in information about other identifiable individuals (e.g., geolocation data). The problem of incidental research subjects is not addressed by the current model of individual control of data through end user license agreements or informed consent.

Emerging Issues for Digital Technologies

The Scale of Data Collection

Mobile devices, ambient listening devices, and other passive data-collection technologies have the capability to collect vast amounts of data with minimal cost and effort, Mello said. There are benefits to this scale of data collection, but there are also concerns. Individual privacy is one such concern, but addressing this concern can raise other issues. For example, allowing surgical patients to opt out of having black box data collected during their procedures could impact quality improvement efforts. Data quality is also a concern, as mobile app users can "fudge" their data in ways that are not generally possible in clinical trials. There are also potential social consequences, such as health care providers stigmatizing or discriminating against noncompliant patients whose behaviors are detected through passive data collection.

The End of Anonymity

The de-identification of data is now recognized to be a temporary state, Mello said. Advances in computer science (e.g., hashing techniques, triangulation of data) have enabled the re-identification of individuals' unlinked data from anonymized datasets. Human research protections are based on the concept that de-identified individual patient data do not present a privacy risk and, therefore, transfers of de-identified data do not require oversight. The increasing potential for re-identification calls for reassessment of this thinking, she suggested.

The Ethical Adolescence of Data Science

Traditional training in science and medicine imparts a set of cultural scientific norms and ethical commitments that may not yet be embedded in the training of computer scientists, Mello said. Digital technology companies currently have a high degree of freedom to self-regulate, yet they may lack a fully formed ethics framework to guide their work. Privacy laws do apply to some degree, though perhaps not to the extent people may think, she added. (The Health Insurance Portability and Accountability Act, for example, does not apply to companies that are not providing health care or supporting health care operations.) There is a need to "establish this profession as a distinct moral community," she said, pointing to the work of Metcalf (2014) and Hand (2018). The field of computer science has developed initial codes of ethics, which she said are a starting point, but more attention is needed.

Next Steps

Some of the ethical concerns associated with emerging digital technologies are new, Mello said, but many are long-standing concerns applied in a new context and with new implications. These ethical concerns cannot be adequately addressed within the existing regulatory system, she concluded. In addition, efforts to address these concerns need to engage people of younger generations and to take into consideration their perspectives on privacy and tradeoffs.

USING ARTIFICIAL INTELLIGENCE AND MACHINE LEARNING IN RESEARCH AND CLINICAL CARE

Artificial Intelligence, Machine Learning, and Bias

The future of AI, Saria said, is in augmenting health care providers' capabilities to more efficiently offer higher-quality care. This includes, for example, reducing diagnostic errors, recognizing diagnoses or complications earlier, targeting therapies more precisely, and avoiding adverse events. Ideally, AI would increase the efficiency of care without increasing the burden on providers.

There has been much discussion and concern about bias in AI algorithms, Saria said. To address these concerns, it is necessary to understand the different underlying problems, but this is hindered by a lack of a taxonomy for understanding bias. Using facial recognition algorithms as an example, Saria discussed six potential errors that could introduce bias.

Inadequate Data

Saria presented a study by Buolamwini and Gebru (2018) that found that the performance of three different facial recognition algorithms in determining gender varied by skin tone. In particular, the algorithms frequently misclassified the gender of darker-skinned females, while the genders of lighter females and both darker and lighter males were classified with much greater accuracy. This weakness, Saria said, is a result of inadequate data. In this case, the underrepresentation of data from specific subpopulations can be addressed by augmenting the data or correcting the algorithms to account for the underrepresentation. Understanding the weakness allows for corrections to be made, but a lack of awareness of the weakness can lead to consequences downstream whose exact nature will depend on how these algorithms are used (e.g., for crime investigation, surveillance, employment).

Asking Bad Questions

Another type of error that can lead to bias is what Saria described as "bad questions." As an example, she described the facial personality profiling offered by a startup technology company. The company claims to use machine learning algorithms for facial analysis to determine traits such as IQ, personality, and career prospects (e.g., whether a person might be a professional poker player or a terrorist). These questions cannot be answered using current observational datasets, Saria said, and there are no experimental interventional datasets in existence to be able to answer these questions. Furthermore, the algorithm is not learning true causal relationships, but rather it is simply mimicking and learning from the data already in the dataset.

Lack of Robustness to Dataset Shift[10]

Error can also be introduced when an algorithm is not robust to dataset shift. To illustrate, Saria described the training and use of a deep learning algorithm for detecting pneumonia in chest X-rays (Zech et al., 2018). The algorithm performed well when used by the same hospital from which the training data were obtained. However, the diagnostic performance deteriorated when the algorithm was then used by a different hospital. This lack of robustness when analyzing datasets from another site, Saria said, was found to be related to style features of the X-rays that varied by institution (e.g., inlaid text or metal tokens visible on the images). This potential source of bias could be corrected by adjusting the algorithm to account for those style features that are not generalizable across datasets.

Evolving Health Care Practice

Provider practice patterns evolve over time, Saria said, and if predictive algorithms are not robust to this type of dataset shift, this can lead to false alerts. As an example, an algorithm for the early detection of sepsis based its predictions on the laboratory tests being ordered by providers and, in

---

[10]Dataset shift is a condition that occurs when data inputs and outputs differ between the training and testing stages. When this occurs, researchers are unable to make generalizations that may allow them to predict events that could occur (Quiñonero-Candela et al., 2009; Subbaswamy et al., 2020).

particular, on whether a measurement of serum lactate level was ordered. The model was trained on data from 2011 through 2013 and performed well when tested in 2014, she said. In 2015, however, predictive performance deteriorated significantly, which Saria explained was associated with a new Centers for Medicare & Medicaid Services requirement for public reporting of sepsis outcomes. As a result of the new regulation, health care institutions increased sepsis surveillance considerably, and laboratory testing for serum lactate levels increased correspondingly. Because the algorithm was not robust to this dataset shift, there were more false alerts.

Model Blind Spots

A small perturbation to a dataset can result in "blind spots" that can lead an algorithm to become "confidently wrong," Saria said. She described a well-known example in which an image, which was correctly identified with confidence by an algorithm as a panda, was minimally perturbed with random noise. Although the change was imperceptible to the human eye and the image appeared to be the same panda, the algorithm determined with high certainly that the image was now a gibbon (Goodfellow et al., 2015). It is important to understand how a learning algorithm is performing so that errors can be addressed, she said.

Human Error in Design

Human error can also lead to bias in models, Saria said. A recent study uncovered bias in an algorithm designed by Optum that is widely used to identify higher-risk patients in need of better care management (Obermeyer et al., 2019). The algorithm was designed to use billing and insurance payment data to predict illness so that high-cost patients could be assigned case managers to help them more proactively manage their health conditions. However, the study found that the high users of health care identified by the algorithm tended to be white, with black individuals using health care less frequently. This resulted in health systems unknowingly offering more care to those already accessing care and thereby further widening the disparities in care.

Addressing Algorithm Biases

A common element across these scenarios, Saria said, is that the errors are generally fixable if the source of the error is known. Changing human behavior is difficult, she said, but point-of-care algorithms, corrected for the sources of bias discussed, can provide "real-time nudges" to influence health care provider decision making.

In developing AI for health care, there is a need for safe and reliable machine learning, Saria said, suggesting that the field could draw from engineering disciplines, which focus on both understanding how a system should behave and then ensuring that it behaves that way. There is excitement about the use of AI in the health care field and interest in downloading and deploying tools, she said, but the underlying "engineering" principles critical for building safe and reliable systems are currently often overlooked (i.e., understanding how these tools work, determining if they are working, and guaranteeing that they continue to work as expected). She described the three pillars of safe and reliable machine learning as failure prevention, failure identification and reliability monitoring, and maintenance. Engineering health care algorithms for safety and reliability involves ensuring that algorithms are more robust to sources of bias (e.g., dataset shift), are able to detect errors (e.g., inadequate data) and identify scenarios or cases that may be outliers in real-time (test-time monitoring), and are updated as needed when shifts or drifts are detected. She referred participants to her tutorial on safe and reliable machine learning for further information (Saria and Subbaswamy, 2019). In closing, Saria suggested that algorithms should be developed, deployed, and monitored post-deployment with the same rigor as prescription drugs (see Coravos et al., 2019).

ETHICAL ISSUES IN MACHINE LEARNING AND DEEP LEARNING NEURAL NETWORKS

Sharing Health Care Data

Many of the ethical issues associated with machine learning involve concerns about data sharing, Ossorio said. There is governance in place for the sharing of research data, and she said that clinical trial participants are becoming increasingly better informed about the ways their data might be shared. However, there is less governance of the sharing of clinical care data. At the federal level there have been efforts to collect and use clinical care data for quality analysis purposes. The training of algorithms requires large amounts of data, which is why, for example, developers such as Alphabet and Microsoft seek to acquire millions of medical images and accompanying medical data from hospital picture archiving and communication systems.

Unlike the case with data collected as part of clinical research, patients interacting with the health care system do not expect their clinical care data to be shared (beyond what is needed to facilitate and coordinate their care). The commercial use of health data currently operates under a very different set of norms, professional commitments, and economic commitments than the clinical research enterprise, Ossorio said, reflecting earlier comments from Mello. While pharmaceutical companies are subject to regulations that protect research participants and the future users of their products, there is not yet comparable oversight of developers of AI for health care. Data are being transferred from the health care context, where the norm is to put the interests of the patient at the center of decision making, to a different context that is not patient-centered.

Price and Cohen (2019) have looked at sharing health data for machine learning, which Ossorio said discusses expanding the "circles of trust" to include entities that develop AI. Whether this should or could be done, given that the norms that govern these types of commercial entities (e.g., Google, Microsoft) are very different from the norms governing clinical research and health care, remains an open question, she said. For example, the norm for development by these types of commercial entities is often to deploy a technology as quickly as possible and then make corrections and updates based on additional data collected while the product is being used in the marketplace. This approach might be acceptable when developing apps that, for example, recommend books or movies for the user. In the health arena, however, drugs and devices generally require premarket assessment of safety and efficacy, she said.

Developing and Implementing Responsible Artificial Intelligence for Health Care

Based on her experience, Ossorio said that many of the companies developing AI do not fully understand the scope or context of health care data. For example, in the case of a machine learning algorithm to aid in the interpretation of clinical laboratory test results, to improve that algorithm after deployment one would need data about how the clinical laboratory is using that test as well as patient clinical outcomes data. However, patient outcomes data generally reside with the health care provider (outcomes data are not usually maintained by the testing laboratory), and the outcomes of interest might appear over the long term. In addition, not understanding the context in which the data were generated can result in the development of an algorithm that is inherently biased or lacks clinical utility.

Another concern, Ossorio continued, is the common perception that those who are expert in developing algorithms can do so using any type of data and that simply providing them with access to volumes of health data will transform the practice of medicine. Collaboration among subject matter experts and algorithm developers is essential for the development and assessment of safe, reliable, useful tools, she said. There is also a need for standards to help ensure the responsible implementation of machine learning algorithms in health care practice (Wiens et al., 2019).

Regulating Machine Learning Algorithms

Algorithms should be held to rigorous standards that are similar to those necessary for the development of drugs, Ossorio said. Most algorithms are not regulated, and those that have been subject to regulation by the U.S. Food and Drug Administration (FDA) thus far have been treated as medical devices. Medical devices generally do not need to meet the same standard of evidence required of drugs before authorization for marketing. The validation of algorithms requires sharing of both code and datasets, Ossorio continued, and researchers are also being encouraged by journals to share code. Because some algorithms are in fact medical devices, Ossorio said, the data used for validation need to be shared according to current regulations and guidelines and need to be labeled as being for research purposes only.

FDA is currently considering how to regulate machine learning algorithms for health care. Algorithms that are cleared or approved by FDA as medical devices are trained, tested, and then locked down prior to implementation, Ossorio said. The challenge now, she said, is how to regulate unlocked or partially unlocked machine learning algorithms that might change over time, perhaps in unpredictable ways.

DISCUSSION

Ethics Training in Data Science and Artificial Intelligence

Are there efforts, Lo asked, to incorporate a discussion of ethical issues into the training of data scientists and AI researchers? Individuals in data science have learned norms and behaviors in the context of the companies they work for and the incentive structures they are presented with, Estrin said, and these do not translate to the health care context. Corrections will require a combination of professional ethics and law, she said. Saria agreed and expressed optimism that positive, corrective action is occurring. All of the leading conferences in the data science field now have discussions of ethics, bias, transparency, and fairness on the agenda, she said, and there are also meetings entirely devoted to these topics. Ossorio was also optimistic and said that, in her experience, data scientists are very interested in discussing ethical issues. Because of this interest she was asked to develop an ethics class for data scientists at her institution, which she said has been popular and is now required for many students in biomedical engineering, biostatistics, public health, and bioinformatics. The curriculum is built around case studies, and she said that engineers and computer scientists have skills in problem solving that translate to solving bioethical problems. A new presidential initiative at Stanford University to provide ethics training to students in computer science has also been very well received, Mello added.

Education on ethical issues in data science is increasing, Estrin said, but the growing interest in ethics in data science should be supported and should also align with laws, regulations, and a shift in incentive structures to help ensure that ethical products can reach the marketplace. Mello said a given field will go through three stages of ethical maturation: recognizing that there are ethical issues, developing a framework for solving those problems, and gaining traction and leadership buy-in so that those who are trained in ethics are supported in taking ethical actions. The field of data science is currently in the first stage, she said, and is just beginning to enter the second.

Transparency and Data Sharing

Transparency in the Absence of Choice

What is the value of transparency, Lo asked, if patients have no choice but to accept sharing of their data as an aspect of receiving services? The health care system where he receives his care, he said, is negotiating the transfer of patient data to a company for algorithm development and validation. Patients do not have a choice about whether their data will be shared, other than to choose not to receive care.

People often feel exploited when they do not feel they have a real choice about sharing their data and do not see a clear benefit of giving up their information, Ossorio said. For example, people might feel they have no choice but to use social media to be informed about work-related information or to stay in touch with family and therefore have no real choice about submitting to the collection and use of their data by the social media websites. They do not perceive that they have made a rational tradeoff of providing information to receive benefits. Transparency about data sharing, even in the absence of choice, she suggested, is better than no transparency because it allows people to engage in political activity to help shape laws and norms. Transparency is also important for building trust. However, transparency is not a solution to deeper ethical problems.

Data Governance

Transparency without data governance is also insufficient, Ossorio said. How data are transferred to the commercial context is important, and license agreements should not lead individuals to relinquish all control. There is a distinction, Estrin said, between institutions selling data and relinquishing responsibility and them collaborating as institutions or providers with companies and bringing their own norms to that collaborative process. This idea, currently part of work being done by her colleagues at Cornell NYC Tech, may be an interesting way to think about data sharing, she added. Many academic institutions have initiated collaborations with for-profit companies, Ossorio said, but full collaboration is often not possible as the digital technology developer is often interested in using the data for an area of research that the data-sharing department or institution does not have interest or expertise in. A challenge, she said, is to define the data governance approach that would be appropriate for that middle ground relationship between a simple transfer of the data and a full research collaboration.

Allowing Patients to Consent or Opt Out of Data Sharing

Should patients be able to opt out of the sharing of their health care data for secondary purposes, Lo asked, and how might that impact the datasets and the ability of researchers to develop and validate digital technologies? Individuals should be given the choice to opt out of data sharing, Saria said, adding that having some patients choose to not share data should not create technical problems for researchers. Institutional infrastructure is the main barrier to implementing an opt-out choice for patients, she said. In her personal experience she has been asked to consent or decline to the sharing of her health data. Whether patients like and trust their providers can influence their decisions on sharing their health data.

There are generational differences in culture and norms that affect the acceptance of information sharing, Saria observed. Generations that grew up using the Internet tend to be more skeptical of what they read online, while older generations are more likely to believe that what they read online is true. Furthermore, she said, she and many others who grew up with the Internet understand and accept that they are receiving services of value to them in exchange for websites collecting and using their user data. Informed consent is important, but there is also a need for education to ensure that people understand what consenting means for them, she said. Many people do perceive data sharing to be exploitative and do not understand or consider the benefits and costs of sharing or not sharing one's data. Institutional leaders who are resistant to providing data to for-profit technology developers at no cost are less concerned about protecting patient privacy, Saria said, and more concerned about not leveraging a potential revenue stream. Instead, they should be thinking about how patients might benefit from more efficient and transparent use of their data.

Estrin agreed that opting out of data sharing should be allowed; however, she said, simply allowing opt outs is not sufficient, and institutions still need to behave responsibly and establish ethical norms, independent of patient choice. Just because a technology or service is provided to consumers at no cost monetarily does not necessarily mean it is acceptable, she added. In many cases it is difficult to avoid a free technology or service because it has become part of the digital technology infrastructure, and in a capitalist economy consumers cannot vote with their purchase power when something is already free.

Unlike patients in integrated health systems, many people do not have the ability to transfer their health data from one provider to another, Estrin noted. Solutions, such as HealthKit (Apple) and CommonHealth (Android), have emerged to allow patients to download their own clinical and health data and to share it across apps and providers. A challenge, she said, is defining which apps or other data users are allowed access to an individual's data. It has been suggested, Estrin said, that consenting to share one's data should be included in the standard terms of service for apps, which advocates say would support frictionless development and innovation by startup companies. However, she said, there is empirical evidence that this type of consent is not sufficient. One option under discussion is that a health system could approve the use of apps that provide some oversight of data sharing and use (i.e., apps that do not sell or reuse patients' data).

Effects of Machine Learning and Artificial Intelligence–Based Tools on Clinician Practice

Is it possible, one workshop participant asked, that physicians might become dependent on digital technology–based interventions that propose interpretations and solutions, and could that dependence degrade provider expertise?

Physician integration with technology is not a new problem, Mello said, and providers have long used different types of decision-support tools (e.g., clinical practice guidelines, automated decision support within the EHR). Questions have been raised as to whether standards are needed for how physicians should interact with digital technologies, she continued, and whether codes of conduct in the medical professions need to address this explicitly. Clinical providers are currently using laboratory tests that employ algorithms for race correction of results (e.g., the calculation of estimated glomerular filtration rate adjusted for race), said a workshop participant. Existing race-based corrections in medicine need to be examined along with new and emerging algorithms, the participant added.

Clinicians and clinical laboratory professionals need training on how to properly use algorithms, Ossorio said. Before that can happen, the algorithms need to be studied to better understand their characteristics and role in practice (e.g., generalizability, indications, contra-indications). These types of studies, however, are not incentivized by the current regulatory system for medical devices, she said.

To what extent, a workshop participant asked, should patients be made aware that provider decisions are being assisted by AI? Providers do not generally discuss with patients the specific resources they use in the course of practice, Mello said, and it is not clear that a patient encounter needs to include discussion of any algorithms used by the provider.

Structural Inequalities in Datasets Used for Algorithm Development

There are structural inequalities embedded in the data being used to develop and train machine learning algorithms, Dorothy Roberts, the George A. Weiss University Professor of Law and Sociology and the director of the Penn Program on Race, Science, and Society at the University of Pennsylvania, said, which can result in the outcomes of predictive analytics being biased (racially biased in particular). Predictive policing, which uses arrest data to predict who in a community is likely to commit crimes in the future, is an example, she said. Discriminatory law enforcement practices (e.g., racially biased stop-and-frisk programs, policing efforts focused on African American neighborhoods) result in racially skewed arrest data that then lead algorithms to predict that those who have the characteristics of black people are likely to commit crimes in the future, she said. There are similar examples in medicine of existing structural inequalities being perpetuated by algorithms, Roberts continued, such as the study of the Optum algorithm discussed by Saria. In that case, an algorithm designed to identify high-risk users of health care in need of additional services was trained using payment data. In choosing health care costs as the dataset, the developers of the algorithm did not take into account the fact that less money is spent caring for black patients, who are often sicker, she said.

Greater collaboration is needed, Roberts said, but that collaboration needs to extend beyond medical professionals and algorithm developers. Collaborations also need to include sociologists and others who understand structural inequality in society and who can recognize errors in datasets that could lead to bias, a point with which Saria agreed.

Structural inequality patterns reflected in datasets can be due to social inequalities that exist outside of the health care system, inequalities in access to health care (e.g., insurance coverage, proximity to providers), and inequalities that have been created within the health care system, Ossorio said. Machine learning algorithms could be helpful in identifying inequalities so that they can be addressed, she suggested; however, assessing the performance of commercial algorithms can be hampered by the fact that these products are frequently licensed—often with restrictions on how they can be studied—rather then sold outright. In some cases, for example, the data used for development are considered a trade secret and are not disclosed.

Potential Research Questions for Funding

Are there research topics in the areas of bioethics, data science, computer science, and digital technology development that should be funded for study? This was the next question Lo posed.

Views on Health Data Sharing and Privacy

Research is needed to better understand how patients would respond if given the choice to opt out of having their clinical data shared with digital technology companies, said Benjamin Wilfond, the director of the Treuman Katz Center for Pediatric Bioethics at Seattle Children's Hospital and Research Institute and a professor in and the chief of the Division of Bioethics and Palliative Care in the Department of Pediatrics at the University of Washington School of Medicine. Mello agreed that how people think through a choice to opt out could be better understood. Studies have used administrative data to assess how many people opt out of programs such as electronic health information exchanges, but these studies do not differentiate between those who have made an informed decision to not opt out (i.e., to participate) and those who simply take no action and participate by default. The role of education in understanding the benefits and risks of participation versus opting out could be studied, she said. It would also be helpful to understand the higher rate of opting out among certain racial and ethnic groups and how the health care enterprise can build trust with these communities. When presented with the choice to opt out, most people will not do anything, Estrin said, so a better question might be how people respond to the choice to opt in (i.e., asking patients to share their data). Most patients presented with an opt-out choice do not fully understand what they are being asked to decide, Saria added. In particular, they do not understand the potential ramifications of not participating (e.g., products of value to them that might not be developed). There is an initiative in the United Kingdom to educate the public about the benefits and risks of sharing or not sharing health data, she said, and this could be a good initiative to replicate in the United States in order to help individuals move from a general fear of data sharing to an understanding of the good that can result.[11] Investment

---

[11]For more information about the United Kingdom's Understanding Patient Data Initiative, see https://understandingpatientdata.org.uk (accessed April 21, 2020).

should go beyond informed consent research to studies of better ways to use data to improve people's lives, she added.

Improving Stakeholder Literacy

Pilot studies could be conducted to explore alternative approaches to individual informed consent, Mello said. Some institutions, for example, have established data use committees to evaluate the proposed uses of health data. Studies could be undertaken to identify the benefits and drawbacks of this approach, compare how the decisions made by the data use committee align with what individuals would choose for themselves, and assess the extent to which committee deliberations reflect the views of minority communities. Understanding intergenerational shifts in perceptions of privacy is another area in need of further research, Mello said. This includes understanding different views on the acceptability of trade-offs (e.g., sharing personal information in return for receiving goods and services at low or no cost). Privacy rules being established now might not be relevant for the next generation, she added. Research could be done, Lo said, to assess patients' understanding of their options regarding data sharing, to identify effective approaches for informing them of their options, and to determine if educating patients about their options changes their behavior.

Research is also needed on how to improve stakeholder literacy, said Camille Nebeker, an associate professor in the University of California, San Diego, School of Medicine. This includes, for example, ensuring that research participants have an adequate understanding of research, data, and technology; that researchers have sufficient literacy in data management; and that students in technology fields gain literacy in ethics. This is an important area for research, Estrin agreed. Developing ethics training programs for computer scientists and educational materials for consumers should not be difficult, Mello said; the challenge is gaining and holding the attention of consumers who are already bombarded with opportunities to consider information and make decisions about data sharing. Ossorio said that an educational approach being developed at Duke provides information about an algorithm in the form of prescribing information (e.g., recommended use, contraindications). This approach quickly and concisely communicates the most important information about an algorithm to users. Research could be done to understand the impact of this and other types of educational interventions on outcomes of interest, Lo suggested.

Assessing Algorithms for Bias and Fairness

Developing metrics and tests that can measure whether an algorithm is biased is another area for research, Saria said. Studies could explore different scenarios in which bias might be present and be used to design tests and metrics to assess the likelihood of bias. Automated approaches to detecting, diagnosing, and correcting bias are needed, she explained, because access to proprietary code and datasets might not be provided, and significant time and resources are needed to conduct in-depth analyses. Metrics are needed for assessing the datasets used for algorithm training, Ossorio agreed, and she noted the importance of understanding the impact of data cleaning on the fairness of datasets. Researchers at the University of Wisconsin have written algorithms that can assess the fairness of other algorithms and can provide input during algorithm training to increase fairness, Ossorio said. This approach is more challenging in the health care context than in many other contexts, she added. There is value in getting researchers and scholars to collaborate in considering different theories of fairness, how they apply in a given context, why one theory might be chosen over another, and how the theories can be built into a software product, she said.

It is also important to learn from the cases of algorithms that did not perform as expected, Estrin said. Working backward to see how the implementation of regulations, laws, or incentives might have altered the outcomes (e.g., prevented the biased outcomes), could be one option, she suggested. In the case of the Optum algorithm discussed by Saria, for example, the company was seeking to optimize patient care in order to control costs. The research question in this case could be, Estrin said, What laws and regulations might have allowed for this optimization function while ensuring ethical outcomes?

Moving Forward

In closing, the panelists reiterated the need for funding to support broad interdisciplinary research in the areas of bioethics and digital technology development. Potential ethical issues need to be addressed up front, Mello said, before digital technologies are released for use, while Estrin underscored the need to understand the incentive structures that currently drive digital technology development and deployment.

3

Ethical Questions Concerning Nontraditional Approaches for Data Collection and Use

Highlights of Key Points Made by Individual Speakers

- Science seeks to understand the world as it is, through logic and observation, but this comes at the cost of embedding the beliefs of those who do the science into descriptions and creations of "facts" and it also lacks any clear linkage to moral issues about how the world "ought" to be in the future. Personal science focuses on understanding the world as it is, like any other science, but incorporates the values, desires, and goals of a person (ought thinking) within scientific discourse. Therefore, personal science might be part of the process needed to bridge "is" and "ought" thinking. Bridging between "is" and "ought" thinking is difficult, but it is necessary to strengthen the trustworthiness of scientific consensus. (Hekler)[1]
- Personal science helps shed light on possible biases that exist and form within professional science. This allows for the opportunity to further address and improve awareness of the issues around biases in the scientific community. (Hekler)
- Those who participate in unregulated personal science often do not have formal training in research practices or ethics. In the new and growing environment of personal science, there is

---

[1] This text was revised after prepublication release.

an opportunity for professional scientists to provide help and guidance to mitigate potential risks. (Nebeker)

- Personal science efforts can raise important questions around power and privilege, including, Who has the right to formulate the questions and to define what qualifies as "success" in personal science? and How can the biomedical research enterprise support individuals in their pursuit of success? (Hekler)
- Persuading individuals to conduct their self-study in an ethical manner involves communicating that an ethical approach to science results in better science and that it is therefore in their own self-interest to engage in personal science in an ethical way. (Wilbanks)
- The freedom to participate in self-study without giving in to surveillance must be structurally built in as people can be coerced into sharing their information and submitting to surveillance. For example, people will often accept free devices and services in exchange for allowing access to their data because this might be their only way to obtain those devices or services. (Wilbanks)

Over the past decade, many new tools for individuals to monitor their own health have emerged, and the public is increasingly engaging in scientific research activities, serving as advocates for their own health. Citizen science (also sometimes referred to as personal science, do-it-yourself science, patient-led research, or participant-led research) is a form of research that takes place outside of the regulatory environment of traditional scientific research,[2] said Camille Nebeker, an associate professor in the University of California (UC), San Diego, School of Medicine, and the session moderator. Originally, citizen scientists partnered with professional scientists to support ongoing research by contributing observations (e.g., counting birds). Community health workers are often engaged as citizen scientists, Nebeker noted, partnering with public health researchers. More recently, individuals have begun conducting their own research without any partnership with professional scientists. Participants in this new system of unregulated personal research may have education in another field and a passion to find a cure for a particular condition, but they have not had training in the practice of scientific research

---

[2]Currently there is not a widely accepted definition of the term "citizen science" (Heigl et al., 2019), but it has been referred to as "the general public engagement in scientific research activities when citizens actively contribute to science either with their intellectual effort or surrounding knowledge or with their tools and resources" (EC, 2014).

or research ethics. "They don't know what they don't know," Nebeker said, and there is the potential for harm.

In this session, Eric Hekler, an associate professor in the Department of Family Medicine and Public Health at UC San Diego, provided an overview of citizen science and discussed what the National Institutes of Health (NIH) could do to advance this area. John Wilbanks, the chief commons officer at Sage Bionetworks, discussed the governance of unregulated research using mobile devices and how individuals engaging in self-study might be persuaded to do so ethically.

CITIZEN AND PERSONAL SCIENCE

Citizen science has been defined by the European Commission as "the general public engagement in scientific research activities," Hekler said (EC, 2014). There are many dimensions to citizen science, including engaging the public in activities related to health research, he said. A subcategory of citizen science is personal science,[3] which has been described as individuals taking a scientific approach to answering questions about their own health and well-being (Heyen, 2020). Individuals might conduct personal research to understand, for example, how they are recovering from a procedure or their response to eating certain foods. As individuals engage in personal science to optimize their health, well-being, or any other personal goal, questions arise about power and privilege, Hekler said. Specifically, who has the right to define what "success" is in personal science, and how can the biomedical research enterprise support individuals in their pursuit of success?

Hekler illustrated examples of citizen science activities based on who is leading the research: citizens, professional scientists, or both as co-developers. These citizen science research activities, he said, can be for the benefit of science, historically marginalized populations, and/or communities and individuals themselves. Who leads the research and who benefits from the research can then be considered against the contribution that the research makes to the health system—whether by enabling overall improved health through activities targeting infrastructure and systems, improving prevention efforts, or improving diagnosis and treatment.

There is great diversity and variation within citizen science activities, Hekler said. Activities vary in terms of who is leading, who it benefits,

---

[3]In Hekler's view, "personal science" can be considered a subcategory of the broader concept of "citizen science." Specifically, if an individual is using the scientific method to support their own goals and desires, they are engaging in personal science. Citizen science is broader and can also involve when individuals take part in research work under the guidance or supervision of others (e.g., bird migration projects).

and the contribution the research makes to the health system. Hekler went on to describe four different types of citizen science activities, beginning with Foldit,[4] a computer game designed by scientists to allow the public to contribute to scientific research on protein folding following an introductory puzzle where players learn what a protein looks like and how to use the game tools to fix common structural issues. Presented with puzzles based on well-understood proteins, the methods in which the puzzles are approached by members of the public are analyzed by researchers in order to improve protein folding software. Propeller Health is another example of a simple digital tool designed by professionals to track a patient's asthmatic symptoms and potential triggers (e.g., pollution).[5] An example of co-development between professionals and citizens is MakerNurse, a collaboration that enables nurses to design, make, and share solutions they develop in the course of providing patient care.[6] Finally, Hekler described OpenAPS, a personal science and patient-led activity that has expanded scientific knowledge and contributed to improved diagnostics and treatment.[7] OpenAPS is an artificial pancreas system designed by Dana Lewis, an individual with type 1 diabetes who is not trained as an engineer or a scientist. Lewis and Scott Leibrand built the system to meet Lewis's own needs and then shared the design for the technology online. There are now more than 2,000 people using similar devices they built using Lewis's open-source specifications. OpenAPS is an example of a personal science activity that has not only helped individual patients but has also contributed to scientific knowledge, spurring peer-reviewed publications and helping to increase the pace of development of artificial pancreas systems, Hekler said.

The Implications of Personal Science

Personal science has implications for professional science and raises questions about what is known and how science is conducted, Hekler said. First, personal science reveals layers of possible biases within professional science. The first layer of possible bias, stereotyping, occurs when individuals are grouped as a research subject or a patient and are essentially told that they should not be taking matters into their own hands and that they should "wait for service" from the scientific research community. The next layer is omission bias. When faced with a potential risk, people tend to favor inaction over action, Hekler said, even when inaction carries the same

---

[4]See https://fold.it/portal (accessed April 15, 2020).
[5]See https://www.propellerhealth.com (accessed April 15, 2020).
[6]See http://makernurse.com (accessed April 15, 2020).
[7]See https://openaps.org (accessed April 15, 2020).

or greater risk. In the clinical research context, essentially asking patients to wait for professional scientific research to provide solutions can result in individual inaction with potential consequences. Furthermore, professionals can be biased toward making sure that solutions are "foolproof" before being released, which could be thought of as a variation of professionals falling into an omission bias. These two variations of the omission bias, occurring both among patients and professionals, could then lead to the last layer—a situation of learned helplessness when people have been told to wait for solutions from the scientific enterprise that never materialize. This can be the case particularly for those with a rare condition that is not a focus of NIH-funded research, Hekler added.

Next, personal science raises questions regarding the process of forming scientific consensus, Hekler said, referring to the work of Boaz Miller, who framed three conditions that can indicate whether there is knowledge-based scientific consensus: calibration (i.e., consensus requires that the parties agree that they want to agree); social diversity; and triangulation of evidence (i.e., having a diversity of methods for generating evidence) (Miller, 2013). The last two, diversity of people and methods, allow for a wide range of knowledge in the process of building trustworthy consensus. If professional science is not hearing from the diversity of voices and methods that personal science brings, it is potentially ignoring valuable information that can promote scientific knowledge, Hekler said.

Finally, personal science asks professional science to "go beyond pure science into 'ought' thinking," Hekler said, drawing from the "is–ought framework" of philosopher David Hume. Professional science sees the world as it is, thinking about science and facts, and focusing on the past and present (which perpetuates systemic biases). A benefit that personal science can bring is that it enables individuals to see and act toward a possible future world or experience as they believe it ought to be. More diverse participation and views in research highlight the need to think further about ethics and morality, along with values and principles, all with an orientation toward the future. Bridging between "is" and "ought" thinking is extremely difficult, Hekler said.

Considerations Moving Forward

Hekler listed four key questions to be addressed in order to start bridging "is" and "ought" thinking and to be considered in future orientation of work and thinking for ethics research moving forward.

- How might professional scientists improve their awareness of systemic implicit biases that, unintentionally, may compromise the capacity to support those served by science?

- How do scientists, unintentionally, compromise equitable participation, contribution, and benefit from the applied sciences? How might scientists improve equity in science?
- How might scientists increase the trustworthiness of scientific consensus, via diversifying the people contributing and diversifying their methods, without compromising their capacity to work toward consensus?
- How do evidence and values interact effectively? How might scientists bridge "is" and "ought" thinking within NIH and beyond?

One way to think about these issues is relative to mechanisms that NIH possesses to potentially strengthen the trustworthiness of scientific consensus and start to bridge "is" and "ought" thinking, Hekler said. Appropriate methods, checklists to define quality, study sections (groups of experts in a given field who review grant applications), and funding opportunity announcements are all mechanisms that work together synergistically. Hekler listed his suggestions for each of the methods and processes.

Methods

Create new and expand on existing NIH-acknowledged best-practice methods in citizen and personal science, keeping emerging open science[8] practices in mind. Open science enables personal science to build upon the work of professional science. For example, the OpenAPS algorithm was built on a commercial continuous glucose monitor and an insulin pump, Hekler explained.

Quality Checklist

Build the appropriate quality checklists that a study section could use to ensure adherence to best-practice methods in citizen and personal science, while not compromising the fundamental epistemological[9] requirements in the approaches taken by self-studies. Evidence-based practice is grounded in clinician experience and prior knowledge. That prior knowledge, however, is grounded in epidemiology, which is population based. Variations of epistemological questions should be considered as a way to add value to self-studies, even though epistemology does not produce generalizable knowledge by itself.

---

[8]The term "open science" can be defined as a set of practices that increase the transparency and accessibility of scientific research (van der Zee and Reich, 2018).

[9]Epistemology involves the philosophical study of how knowledge is acquired and disseminated.

Study Sections

Create new study sections filled with a diversity of citizen and personal scientists along with traditional professionals who, together, support rigor in this type of science. Professionals from sociology and the humanities, who have a long history and tradition of studying and understanding structural biases, should be included.

Funding Opportunity Announcements

Create funding opportunity announcements that legitimize and fund a wider range of contributors (e.g., participant-led work) and methods.

In closing, Hekler reminded participants that article 27 of the Universal Declaration of Human Rights states that "Everyone has the right to participate ... [and] share in scientific advancements and its benefits,"[10] which is increasingly becoming a rallying cry from leaders in advancing personal science.

GOVERNANCE OF UNREGULATED HEALTH RESEARCH USING MOBILE DEVICES

Today's smartphones have far greater capabilities than simply spoken communication, Wilbanks said. A typical iPhone, for instance, has facial recognition technology, a barometer, a three-axis gyroscope, an accelerometer, a proximity sensor, and an ambient light sensor. And individuals today have access to many other advanced technologies beyond the smartphone. On the retail website Alibaba, one can purchase an electroencephalograph, a pulse oximeter, and other medical devices at a relatively low cost. Due to the advantages in the affordability and availability of these types of materials and devices, the research capabilities in personal science are accelerating quickly.

Wilbanks and colleagues set out to examine potential ethical and policy questions related to unregulated health research using mobile devices in the United States. Specifically, the study addressed how independent individuals and entities pursuing self-led research could be influenced to do what is ethically right when they are not legally obligated to do so and might not agree that it is necessary. With funding from NIH,[11] Wilbanks

---

[10]See https://www.un.org/en/universal-declaration-human-rights (accessed April 15, 2020).

[11]Addressing ELSI Issues in Unregulated Health Research Using Mobile Devices, No. 1R01CA20738-01A1, National Cancer Institute, National Human Genome Research Institute, and Office of Science Policy and Office of Behavioral and Social Sciences Research in the Office of the Director, National Institutes of Health, Mark A. Rothstein and John T. Wilbanks, Principal Investigators.

and colleagues conducted a series of qualitative interviews with thought leaders including application (app) and device developers, researchers using mobile devices, patient and research participant advocates, and regulatory and policy professionals. Four working group meetings were also convened to gather input from stakeholders. The findings and recommendations were published in a special issue of *The Journal of Law, Medicine & Ethics* and were disseminated to app developers and policy makers at two workshops (Rothstein et al., 2020).

Preventing Harms from Unregulated Health Research Using Mobile Devices

A range of options for preventing harms from unregulated health research using mobile devices were offered by the members of the working group. One option considered was to extend the Common Rule to apply to all research and all researchers.[12] The Common Rule was designed to safeguard the welfare and interests of research participants and society. Although the vast majority of other countries use the approach of extending the Common Rule, Wilbanks said there is little political support for taking this approach in the United States. Another option proposed within the working group was to maintain the status quo. The supporting arguments for not taking any action were that there have not been any adverse consequences thus far and that regulation could drive research underground or result in some valuable research not being done. In the end, neither of these options was considered to be practical.

Instead, the research group focused on approaches to persuading people to conduct their self-study in an ethical manner. Steps defined included establishing outer boundaries, providing education and assistance, and appealing to their self-interest and their sense of decency. The approach focuses on communicating to individuals that an ethical approach to science results in better science and that it is therefore in an individual's own self-interest to engage in personal science in an ethical way.

Potential Opportunities for Various Stakeholders

The study report details the investigators' recommendations for action by states, NIH, the U.S. Food and Drug Administration (FDA), the Federal Trade Commission (FTC) and the Consumer Product Safety Commission (CPSC), the Centers for Disease Control and Prevention (CDC), consumer

---

[12]For information on the Federal Policy for the Protection of Human Subjects, known as the Common Rule, see https://www.hhs.gov/ohrp/regulations-and-policy/regulations/common-rule/index.html (accessed April 15, 2020).

technology companies (including app stores), and individual unregulated researchers (e.g., citizen scientists, do-it-yourself researchers). Wilbanks highlighted several of the top-level recommendations from the study in each area (see Rothstein et al., 2020).

- **States** can take action in the absence of federal laws and regulations. Wilbanks cited the state research law enacted by Maryland as an example.[13] This law broadly defines "person performing research" and requires that those persons conform to the Common Rule.
- **NIH** has the ability and the opportunity to educate and assist unregulated researchers in conducting ethical self-research. One recommendation from the study, Wilbanks said, is for NIH to establish an Office of Unregulated Health Research to provide more accessible information regarding ethical practices for self-research. NIH cannot fund unregulated research studies, but it can fund studies about unregulated research to elucidate the actual risks and benefits.
- **FDA** only regulates mobile apps that function as medical devices and that could pose a risk to patient safety if they fail to function as intended, Wilbanks said. However, there are ongoing interagency collaborative efforts to reduce regulatory duplication and identify areas unaddressed by current regulation that the study recommended be continued. Wilbanks added that the health app developer and health device developer communities are closely watching the regulatory environment, and he said the threat of FDA regulation is a powerful incentive that could be put to better use.
- **FTC** has the potential to play a greater role in the area of consumer protection, Wilbanks said. **CPSC** has influence over the types of products that are marketed and the claims that are made about products. The study recommended that FTC make targeted enforcement actions against developers of unregulated mobile research applications who engage in deceptive or unfair trade practices, Wilbanks said. The study also recommended that FTC increase monitoring of the security of and improve the security practices of the hardware and software components of tools for self-research. He noted that software security vulnerabilities are often propagated by developers who simply copy and paste bad security source code shared by others.
- **CDC** expertise in epidemiological surveillance could be extended to surveillance for security vulnerabilities related to mobile health research tools. The sharing of flawed code can create vulnerabilities

---

[13]Md. Code Ann., Health-Gen. §§ 13-2001–2002.

that can promote misinformation and allow for leakage of personal information, Wilbanks said. The study recommended that CDC work with NIH and private entities to understand the scope of the issue and to establish a system to monitor trends in security vulnerabilities over time.

- **App stores,** such as those maintained by Apple and Google, are powerful de facto regulators of which products reach consumers' mobile devices and computers, Wilbanks said. For example, Apple requires apps developed with ResearchKit to secure approval by an institutional review board (IRB). The study recommended that Google implement a comparable policy and that both companies require developers to upload the IRB approval letter and make it available to consumers. App stores could also prioritize where apps appear in search results based on adherence to certain norms, require that terms of service and privacy policies for health apps explicitly ban third-party data transfer, and require device developers to encrypt data both at rest and in transit.
- **Citizen science organizations** reach unregulated researchers through social media, meet-ups, and mailing lists, and Wilbanks said these groups need to be better leveraged to promote ethical self-research. Often, these groups are only engaged when they are being "scolded." One study recommendation calls for these organizations to create guidance for their members on how to transparently communicate the goals, risks, and benefits of their research.

DISCUSSION

To open the discussion, Nebeker described Quantified Self as another example of a citizen science organization.[14] Quantified Self is a community of people supporting one another in the conduct of self-study. In some cases individuals engaging in self-study are living with a significant health problem that they feel the health system is not addressing sufficiently, Nebeker said. In other cases, individuals might be looking to improve personal well-being or performance (e.g., better sleep patterns, faster marathon time).

Nebeker provided research ethics guidance to a Quantified Self participant-led research project to study personal daily lipid levels. The leaders were interested in thinking through study risks, benefits, and risk-management solutions. Because this was a group of individuals engaging in self-study to gain individual knowledge, the project did not meet the federal definition of human subjects research as it was not considered to be "generalizable knowledge," which is a classifier for defining research

---

[14]See https://quantifiedself.com (accessed April 15, 2020).

subject to the Common Rule or IRB review, she explained. However, the group did publish a discussion of the process of conducting responsible and safe participant-led research (Grant et al., 2019). In this participant-led research, participants studied their daily lipid levels over time, and each of these single-subject studies led to observations that the leaders wanted to share via a peer-reviewed publication. For consideration of this manuscript, the publisher requested IRB approval documentation. Because an IRB was not involved prospectively (because the study did not meet the definition of research with human subjects), the group "worked the system" and requested an IRB to declare the study as exempt from IRB review as it involved existing data, Nebeker said. This is not ideal, as the federal definitions within the Common Rule do not speak to self-study or self-experimentation, and yet journals are bound by the traditional conventions requiring research involving humans to obtain an IRB approval, which leads to the question of how to better support the responsible and ethical conduct of self-study.

Power and Privilege in Citizen and Personal Science

Acknowledging and Balancing the Power Differential

Hekler drew from his own experience to discuss further the gaps in power and privilege in citizen and personal science. He spoke about how he first met Lewis when she was giving a talk at a conference about her OpenAPS project. He was very interested in the project and offered to help by conducting a clinical efficacy trial. Lewis politely declined, and Hekler realized that he had made the mistake of assuming he knew what he could do to help. This is an example of the psychological bias called the Dunning–Kruger effect, which, he said, could be summarized as "confident ignorance."

Afterward, Hekler and Lewis together identified the way in which he could contribute, and they applied for and were awarded a grant from the Robert Wood Johnson Foundation to study how to open pathways to innovation for citizen scientists. During the planning for this grant, Hekler said he began assuming the role of principal investigator (PI) for the study because he has training as a PI. However, he and Lewis came to realize again that this was Lewis's study and that she should fulfill the role of PI. As part of the study, traditional and nontraditional experts were convened to discuss opening pathways for innovation and to specifically consider the issues of power and privilege. Another learning experience for Hekler was being assigned by Lewis to be a nonparticipating note-taker for the entire workshop. Although, at first he felt that he was better suited to help synthesize the group outcome, he said, he came to realize that contributing from his perspective as a white male of privilege would have compromised the desire for equitable participation from all who can, particularly non-traditional patient scientists. He said that he now tries to be conscious about the impact of gaps in power and privilege when working with citizen-led research projects.

It is critical to understand and address issues of power and privilege, Hekler said. There are implicit biases and structural forces that assign status to people. It is not enough to invite particular individuals to participate (i.e., tokenism), he said. The environment must be such that these people also feel comfortable and safe in participating. Furthermore, he said, those who traditionally hold power (e.g., professional researchers) need to recognize when they are falling into the trap of confident ignorance and emotional blindness (i.e., never having experienced that which someone else is describing and thus not being able to relate and truly understand).

Self as Subject

The principle of respect for persons participating in research is embodied in the informed consent process, Nebeker said. The challenge is to ensure that same respect for persons in a self-study. How does an individual consent himself or herself? For the Quantified Self participant-led study, which involved the collection of blood via finger prick, she said that an explicit process was developed to help self-researchers through the decision-making process, considering both the potential risks and the benefits. She noted that even though each person was conducting self-study, there was the potential for outside influence (e.g., not wanting to disappoint others in the group).

Hekler said that the question underlying self-study is who has the power and privilege to be able to ask the questions and define success. For example, he said that Lewis and Leibrand have the capacity to develop OpenAPS (e.g., time, resources, education, a network). Acknowledging this power and privilege, Lewis's intention in securing the grant from the Robert Wood Johnson Foundation was to enable pathways to innovation for others, Hekler said. There are many examples of approaches to building the context and the capacity that can enable individuals to use research to support their personal needs, Hekler said (e.g., community-based participatory research partnerships, youth participatory action research networks, and initiatives such as the Patient-Centered Outcomes Research Institute).

Structural Inequalities

Structural inequalities prevent many people from engaging in self-research. Too often the institutional reaction is to solve the problem for those affected, Hekler said. But there are often unintended consequences resulting from a lack of understanding of the context (e.g., food aid provided to developing countries can adversely affect local economies and perpetuate food insecurity). Instead, initiatives should focus on building the capacity for people to ask the research questions that are relevant to their own context and lived experiences and, ultimately, solve their own issues, with advice, support, and plausible solutions that worked elsewhere provided by professionals.

Institutions are not supporting citizens who want to better understand their own lives in the context of their health, Nebeker said. She recalled an example from her own institution in which one of her students who was interested in studying her own pain designed a self-study and approached the university IRB for approval. The IRB's context for self-study was limited to that of university physicians or researchers studying themselves, Nebeker said. The members of the IRB had no understanding of why a student would want or need to conduct a self-study, and they advised her against it. This example is indicative of the regulatory definitions found in the Common Rule limiting the ability of people doing self-study to seek an external review. With the growth of citizen science applied to health, this is an area that NIH could help to guide by supporting research on developing relevant infrastructures.

Wilbanks described how structural issues could lead to people essentially being coerced into sharing their information and submitting to surveillance, sometimes for ethically questionable purposes. Those who can afford the latest technology devices can choose to engage in self-study that is relatively ethical and free of surveillance, he said. Others will often accept free devices and service in exchange for allowing access to their data because this is a way to obtain desirable devices that they would not otherwise be able to get. As an example, he said that the Apple Heart Study offered individuals who agreed to participate the opportunity to obtain Apple watches at a subsidized price. The freedom to participate in self-study without giving in to surveillance must be structurally built in, Wilbanks said.

The National Institutes of Health's Role in Guiding Unregulated Research

Nebeker asked the other panelists to expand on how NIH might work with citizen science and personal science organizations to guide unregulated research. Wilbanks offered several potential areas where NIH could focus.

Education

NIH should invest in educating citizen and personal scientists on clinical research, Wilbanks said. People need to understand that there is a process of gathering data, analyzing data, and drawing conclusions and that scientific conclusions are not truths but rather are claims that "exist at varying degrees of truth over time."

Clarify the Application of the Common Rule to Research Supported by Indirect Funding

Many institutions in the United States believe that only direct funding is covered by the Common Rule, Wilbanks said. Citizen science organizations question why their members should follow the Common Rule when they are aware of institutions that claim that their research supported by indirect funding is not covered by the Common Rule. A clarifying statement from NIH would be helpful, he said.

Engage the Citizen Scientist Community as Equals

Feedback from the citizen and personal science community has revealed that they have often felt unwelcome and disregarded by the institutional science community, Wilbanks said. He urged NIH to create opportunities for the institutional, citizen, and personal science communities to meet as equals and learn from each other. He suggested attending citizen science association meetings and hearing their critiques and concerns.

Create Safe Harbors for Data-Hosting Platforms

Safe harbors are needed for data-sharing platforms, Wilbanks said. Although Internet platforms are not liable for copyright infringement resulting from information posted by users, there are no such protections for data hosting platforms. Data-hosting platforms that are trying to do the right thing can still be held liable in the event of a failure—and to the same extent as a malicious actor, he said. Legislating a safe harbor for data-hosting platforms that limits damages would be helpful, he said, although he acknowledged that this is not likely to be a priority for Congress in the near future.

Oversight Systems: Principles Versus Processes

Developing and evaluating different systems of oversight that could be applied to both citizen science and mobile health could be an area for NIH to consider funding, Wilbanks suggested. What is needed is not more principles of bioethics, Nebeker said, but rather practices that evolve with the changing ecosystem. She said that the community needs to be engaged, more authentically and more frequently, in discussions about shaping the future of citizen science and self-study. Patients and the public have not been asked about their understanding of their data, of who wants to access their data, or of what can be learned from their data. To apply the principle of justice it is necessary to consider who is being included and excluded and who stands to benefit, she said.

The principles of bioethics are being confused with the process of bioethics, Wilbanks said. He agreed with Nebeker that the principles are sound, but he said that specific institutional processes might not meaningfully reflect those principles. For example, the objectives of researchers have become to get IRB approval and then consent and enroll patients into a study, not necessarily to meaningfully think about the risks and benefits of a study and then to meaningfully inform potential participants about them. NIH should reinforce the principles and develop new processes and practices that implement them, he added. Hekler suggested an organizational structure for facilitating oversight of the implementation of ethical principles. Rather than a centralized structure or one composed of subgroups, he proposed a resilient, diverse network of different groups with different powers that allows for checks and balances, much like the logic of the U.S. Constitution. The first step, he said, will be to understand how to balance those powers in the face of systemic biases.

4

Understanding the Impact of Inequality on Health, Disease, and Who Participates in Research

Highlights of Key Points Made by Individual Speakers

- The numerous inequities that are apparent across racial groups are the result of structural inequalities and racism. It is important to differentiate between research designed to identify innate biological differences in people who are disadvantaged by social inequality (in the hope of developing a therapy), and research studying how inequitable structures are embodied by people (and then addressing those structures). (Roberts)
- More diverse stakeholder engagement in the discussions about research ethics is needed before a more diverse population can be expected to participate in research. This will require investment in research on the effects of inequitable structures on health, including those that reinforce inequalities based on race, socioeconomic status, gender, and disability, among others. (Roberts)
- For federally recognized American Indian/Alaska Native tribes, the right to self-determination includes authority over how and what type of research may be conducted within tribal communities. Studies should be in alignment with tribal priorities and the values of the community, and core principles of respect and reciprocity must be adhered to when asking research questions. (Hiratsuka)

> • Current national policies regarding study review and approval, participant recruitment and consent, return of results, and data sharing, storage, and stewardship might not align with tribal sovereignty rights and values. (Hiratsuka)

Inequalities can be based on race, gender, national origin, language, sexual orientation, disability, veteran status, and any number of other characteristics, said Anita Allen of the University of Pennsylvania. In this session, panelists considered the impact of inequality on health, disease, and who participates in research. Dorothy Roberts, the George A. Weiss University Professor of Law and Sociology and the director of the Penn Program on Race, Science, and Society at the University of Pennsylvania, discussed the ethical and structural issues related to the relationship between race and racism. Vanessa Hiratsuka, a senior researcher at Southcentral Foundation, discussed bioethical issues that are unique to American Indian and Alaska Native tribes due to their status as both a racial group and a political entity. The session was moderated by Allen.

THINKING ETHICALLY AND STRUCTURALLY ABOUT RACE AND RACISM

One of the central bioethical questions is about the relationship between social inequalities and biology, Roberts said. The idea that social inequalities are caused by innate biological differences (e.g., race, gender) has long been used to justify the unethical and abusive treatment of groups of people. This argument was used to rationalize the enslavement of black people by white people, for example. The eugenics movement was also based on the false idea that heritable, innate traits were the root of social inequalities. "Inequalities of power based on race have been blamed on innate biological differences between races," Roberts said, and for this session she focused her remarks on the idea that "race is a scientific invention."

The Origins of Race

Roberts reminded participants that the major categories of race used today derive from the racial typology defined by anthropologist Johann Blumenbach in the late 1700s and that the work of historian Terence Keel suggests that the Enlightenment sciences adopted the idea that human beings are naturally divided into races from Christian theology. Furthermore, she said, the conduct of science has been influenced significantly since then by the invention of racial categories. Even today, scientific studies involving human participants routinely categorize them into supposedly biological races, though researchers typically use social groupings. Roberts said that the impact of applying this concept of biological race to the fundamental design and conduct of science has not yet been fully explored. "Racism is not the product of race," Roberts emphasized, but rather "race is the product of racism." The idea that certain groups of people are naturally entitled to dominate other groups came first, she said. Accepting that idea then required the political division of people into races both to govern unequal societies and to pretend that social inequality is natural. She suggested keeping in mind that racism necessitates the invention of race when considering scientific questions.

Structural Racism

Structural racism is a significant contributor to racial inequalities in health. As an example, Roberts noted that the maternal mortality rate in the United States has been steadily rising, in contrast to nearly all other developed countries and even many developing countries, where it is declining. Furthermore, she said, black women are three to four times more likely than white women to die from pregnancy-related causes. Evidence of the role of structural inequalities in this disparity abounds, yet research continues to look for innate biological characteristics to explain the higher rates of black maternal mortality as well as black infant mortality.

To illustrate, she cited a peer-reviewed journal article that described a study of the role of "black race independent of other factors" in pre-term birth (Kistka et al., 2007). The hypothesis of the study presumes to strip away all social determinants of health and test some essence of black race as the cause of the increased risk of pre-term births. In addition to the study's failure to define "black race" or to control for all significant social determinants, the central flaw with such hypotheses is that race itself is not a risk factor and should never be treated as such, Roberts said. Racism, however, is a risk factor, and the numerous inequities that are apparent across racial groups are the result of structural inequalities and racism, she said.

The Embodiment of Racism

It is important to recognize, Roberts said, quoting her own work, that "race is not a biological category that naturally produces health disparities because of genetic differences. Race is a political category that has staggering biological consequences because of the impact of social inequality on people's health" (Roberts, 2018, p. 129). This claim is based on an increasing body of research on the ways in which racism is embodied. She highlighted an opinion piece from *The New York Times* titled "We're Sick of Racism, Literally" and said there are many studies now on this topic.[1]

Roberts urged researchers to study how inequitable structures are embodied by individuals and groups—and then to address those structures—rather than focusing on innate biological differences and biological interventions. The Tuskegee syphilis experiment[2] is often cited as one of the reasons why black people are often reluctant to participate in clinical research, Roberts said, but people are also reluctant to participate in research that is geared toward "fixing them" rather than addressing the underlying social structures that they know are harming their health.

Promoting Structural Change

To make societal structural change a reality, it will be necessary to understand who has an investment in keeping things the way they are and who is invested in changing society, Roberts said. Those who are socially disadvantaged have the greatest stake in structural change, she said, and it is therefore important that they be included in discussions of bioethics in research. In contrast, those conducting the research typically have little stake in structural change and, in fact, often benefit from preserving the status quo. Roberts mentioned the current discussions of the bioethics of gene editing as an example. Those engaged in gene-editing research have a greater stake in promoting genetic enhancement as a method to improve the human condition, she said, and less of a stake in promoting societal change. More diverse and meaningful stakeholder engagement in discussions about research ethics and the research agenda is needed before a more diverse population can be expected to participate in research, she concluded.

FEDERAL INDIAN LAW AND BIOETHICS

To start her presentation, Hiratsuka noted that the workshop was taking place on the ancestral lands of the Anacostans, also documented as the Nacotchtank. The District of Columbia and surrounding areas in Maryland and Virginia along the Anacostia and Potomac Rivers were once home to many sovereign indigenous peoples, including the Piscataway, the

---

[1]See https://www.nytimes.com/2017/11/11/opinion/sunday/sick-of-racism-literally.html (accessed April 15, 2020).

[2]The Tuskegee syphilis experiment refers to an unethical clinical study (Tuskegee Study of Untreated Syphilis in the Negro Male) carried out from 1932–1972 by the U.S. Public Health Service. The goal of the study was to understand the natural history of untreated syphilis; however, the African American men involved in the study did not receive accurate information about the risks associated with the study. Researchers also withheld penicillin from participants.

Pamunkey, the Nentego also known as the Nanichoke, the Mattaponi, the Chickahominy, the Monacan, the Powhatan, and the Patawomeck. Indigenous people in the District of Columbia area continue to fight for federal government recognition of their nations and the right to establish a government-to-government relationship with the United States, Hiratsuka said. Hiratsuka is a member of the Navajo Nation, one of the largest tribes in both population and physical size, and is also of the Winnemem Wintu, a tribe whose legal rights were terminated.

The Federal Regulation of American Indians and Alaska Natives

The peoples of the American Indian and Alaska Native tribes are recognized as both a racial group and a political entity. The American Indian/ Alaska Native populations face many of the same bioethical issues discussed thus far at the workshop, but there are also some unique concerns that stem from the political designation of these populations, Hiratsuka said.

There are currently 574 tribes officially listed as "Indian entities recognized and eligible to receive services from the United States Bureau of Indian Affairs," Hiratsuka said.[3] Of those, 231 are Alaska Native tribes. The U.S. Constitution recognizes these American Indian tribes as sovereign nations with the right to self-determination and grants Congress the authority to interact with Indian tribes. The right to self-determination includes authority over how and what type of research may be conducted within tribal communities, Hiratsuka said.

The application of federal Indian law can subject American Indian/ Alaska Native people to extensive legal regulation of their rights, Hiratsuka said, and she cautioned that "what can be granted, can be taken away." For example, tribes have had their recognition terminated, their rights to ancestral lands and to engaging in cultural practices denied, and their access to sacred lands and waters prevented. Tribes have also been prohibited from exercising their tribal authority over non-members in land-use situations, from resolving criminal violations committed by Indians on Indian land, and from prosecuting non-Indians who commit crimes on Indian land.

American Indian/Alaska Native Health and Health Care

As a group, American Indian/Alaska Native people have experienced "deliberate and intentional historical trauma," Hiratsuka said, and their collective psychological injury spans generations. Assimilation policies and programs separated American Indian/Alaska Native people from their families and tribes and denied them access to sacred lands and cultural practices.

---

[3] As of February 19, 2020.

Historically and to this day, American Indian/Alaska Native people experience significant health disparities relative to the general population and to other minority populations.[4]

Health care services have been provided to tribes through federally funded organizations, previously through the Department of War and now through the Indian Health Service of the U.S. Department of Health and Human Services. In addition, the Indian Self-Determination and Education Assistance Act of 1975 allows for direct funding of tribes to deliver health care services themselves. The tribally administered health programs have been very successful in improving the health of the population, Hiratsuka said, and they provide another avenue to care besides the Indian Health Service, which she described as chronically underfunded. Provisions of the Indian Health Care Improvement Act address improving current health care services, increasing the services available to urban-dwelling American Indian/Alaska Native people, and promoting the education and retention of health professionals to work in tribal communities.

Research Bioethics

"The path from research to tribal health benefit is long and uncertain," Hiratsuka said. American Indian/Alaska Native people have faced a range of bioethical transgressions when engaging with the research community, social scientists, and clinical services. These include the failure to be inclusive and transparent, the failure to share the results and the benefits of research, and the failure to protect group and individual rights and confidentiality. Tribal populations that are small and have unique genetic profiles are at increased risk for community identification and stigmatization, she noted. It is also important, Hiratsuka said, to recognize that current national policies regarding study review and approval, participant recruitment and consent, the return of results, and data sharing, storage, and stewardship might not align with tribal sovereignty rights and values.

As a result of these and other ethical failures and harms, members of the American Indian/Alaska Native community remain skeptical about engaging in research. For example, she said, there are concerns about comprehensive, long-term data collection, such as that being done as part of the National Institutes of Health (NIH) All of Us Research Program,[5] particularly how tribal members' data could be misused. Tribal communities

---

[4]More information about health disparities in the American Indian and Alaska Native tribes can be found at https://www.ihs.gov/newsroom/factsheets/disparities (accessed April 21, 2020).

[5]The All of Us Research Program is working to create a database for health research by collecting data from 1 million people living in the United States. See https://allofus.nih.gov (accessed April 15, 2020)

are deliberating about whether and how to engage in research, including how best to operationalize respect for both tribal authority and individual autonomy and how to prevent both individual physical harm and group harms.

Southcentral Foundation has been conducting health research, Hiratsuka said, and in her experience, the Alaska Native people are interested in and see benefits in participating. Ongoing community engagement is required, she said, and the research must be conducted under the authority of the tribal nations. Before any research can be done, the organization and the tribal leadership work together to develop an additional process, a community-level review of the research, to ensure that the studies are in alignment with tribal priorities and the values of the community. Because of this, she said, some practices that are standard elsewhere might not be done (e.g., non-tiered broad consent, storage of specimens in national repositories, documentation of pedigrees, genome-wide sequencing). The use of stigmatizing language needs to be avoided, and pre-publication tribal review of manuscripts is also important, she added.

DISCUSSION

Researcher Awareness and Attention to Structural Inequities

Panelists were asked by Anita Allen, the session moderator, to speak about the extent to which researchers understand the impacts of inequality (economic, social), discrimination, and racism on health and disease and what steps could be taken to improve their understanding. For hundreds of years and until relatively recently, the prevailing view in science was that social inequalities in health were caused by innate biological defects, Roberts reiterated. It was the view of a small minority that social conditions were at the root of unequal health outcomes along social lines, she said. This was articulated by W. E. B. Du Bois in his study *The Philadelphia Negro* (Du Bois, 1899). Du Bois concluded that the reason black people suffered from poor health was political and resulted from their being forced to live in the slums of Philadelphia, Roberts said. Du Bois believed the poor health of black people was not because their bodies could not adapt to freedom or that they were biologically suited to be enslaved. Du Bois also pointed out that the Irish were once thought to be predisposed to consumption (tuberculosis) when they were "unpopular."

Only recently has research been specifically targeted to understanding how social inequalities are embodied, Roberts said. Research has focused on the role of neighborhood segregation in increased risk for poor health. For example, segregated black and brown neighborhoods are more likely to be in close proximity to highways and to have greater exposure to toxins, such as lead. Research on epigenetics has begun to elucidate the impact of unequal environments, including social environments, on gene expression. Studies have demonstrated that states with higher rates of structural inequality also have a higher rate of heart attacks among black people. Researchers are also studying how exposure to police killings of unarmed black people affects health in the community. Roberts suggested that more funding should be directed toward this important new area of research that examines the effect of structural inequalities on health.

Even in the face of this emerging research, Roberts said, many researchers are still drawn to looking for innate biological explanations of societal differences in health in the hope of developing pharmaceutical or biological cures. Ultimately, study participants know that their health is associated with their structural conditions, but proposals for change in these conditions are rarely generated from these studies. She suggested that more research funding is needed to study the health impacts of policies that address structural inequities. For example, studies have shown the associations between racially disparate arrests of teenagers and poor health outcomes. However, Roberts observed that proposed solutions tend to focus on intervening in the bodies or behaviors of black teenagers, whereas it is often considered unscientific, biased, or inappropriate to propose and study ways to stop police from disproportionately arresting them. A better understanding is needed of how economic, racial, gender, disability, and other inequalities cause poor health outcomes, she concluded, and researchers need to think more broadly about scientific solutions to structural inequities.

Researcher Awareness and Attention to Study Population Worldview

Hiratsuka recalled Hekler's discussion of power and privilege (see Chapter 3) and his discomfort with being present and observing but not engaging. Minority populations often feel that although they are invited to be present, they are not asked to engage, she said. Hiratsuka mentioned the phrase "not about us without us" and said that American Indian and Alaska Native populations are very interested in engaging in the discussions on who gets to ask the questions, who is conducting the research, what data are being collected, and how those data will be used.

Collaboration with the community is essential for researchers to understand the context in which American Indian/Alaska Native community members live, Hiratsuka said. Few researchers have had the same lived experience as the people from minority communities they are working to serve. For example, does a researcher seeking to develop interventions for diabetes understand that some healthy foods that might be recommended are at odds with traditional foods? The core principles of respect and reciprocity must be adhered to when asking research questions, Hiratsuka said. "What is benefit and who determines benefit, what is harm and who determines harm?" Researchers need to be comfortable letting go, she said, and letting others ask and respond to these questions.

The National Institutes of Health's All of Us Research Program

Allen asked panelists for their perspectives on the NIH All of Us Research Program. It is important to understand why people are being enrolled according to certain racial or ethnic criteria, Roberts responded. If the goal of a project is to enroll a more racially diverse population, then what meaning of race is being used, she asked, and what are the assumptions about how this diversity would change the project? She noted that there are reasons for enrolling more people of underrepresented races in clinical research that are not based on assumed biological differences between races. One reason could be to extend the benefits of clinical research participation more equitably to a broader group of people. Another reason is to expand the overall diversity of the study population broadly relative to biology, geography, physical characteristics, or other aspects (i.e., not based on an idea that each race is a biologically homogeneous group of people with a particular set of traits).

Roberts noted a concern about the potential uses of any genetic material that is collected. It is not uncommon for DNA collected for one purpose to be used for another purpose entirely, she observed. Selling samples to for-profit companies or sharing them with law enforcement opens up the possibility for discrimination by state or private actors, she said.

Hiratsuka also raised concerns about the purpose and repurpose of the various data types collected as part of the All of Us Research Program. For example, it is not clear who is reviewing and approving research projects on behalf of members of tribal communities or how the interests of tribal communities can be protected when the potential research uses are unclear or without distinct purpose, she said. There is particular concern that a tribal consultation process was not instituted prior to the start of data collection for the project,[6] especially given that the goal of the project is to enroll a diverse population, she noted.

Diversity of socioeconomic status is often absent from research initiatives, including the All of Us Research Program, a workshop participant noted, even though the data indicate socioeconomic status is an important determinant of health. One reason that socioeconomic status might not be

---

[6]More information about current efforts in the All of Us Research Program to engage and consult with tribal leaders from the American Indian and Alaska Native communities can be found at https://allofus.nih.gov/about/diversity-and-inclusion/all-us-tribal-engagement (accessed May 19, 2020).

included, Roberts suggested, is because if one rejects the idea that inequities in socioeconomic status are produced by innate biological differences but also believes individual heath is determined primarily by genes, then there would seem to be no reason to include socioeconomic status in the study (i.e., if socioeconomic status is not caused by innate differences, then it is irrelevant to health). Such thinking reflects the assumption that any kind of health problem must stem from innate causes. Roberts expressed concern that the All of Us Research Program is focused too much on the belief that more genetic knowledge is the answer to health problems and inequities.

Terminology Choices Perpetuate Assumptions

The terminology used in the workshop title, "Bioethical Issues in Bio-medical Research," implies that biology is a key determining factor for health, noted a workshop participant. The tools of health are most often pharmaceuticals and medical devices, not approaches to address underly-ing social determinants of health, the participant said. It is challenging to find the right terminology that includes the social element equally with the biological and acknowledges that human beings do not exist apart from society, Roberts said. Hiratsuka also commented on the use of "emerging" in relation to bioethical issues in the workshop title. These ethical ques-tions have been discussed for decades within communities that experience considerable inequalities, she said.

Groups Needing Additional Representation

A workshop participant agreed with Hiratsuka about the important role of the tribal authority in helping determine whether research should go forward. These bodies complement the work of institutional review boards to ensure that individuals are able to make informed choices about participation and also help to protect the interests of the larger group. As an example, samples preserved from Tay-Sachs research done in the early 1970s were later used for the early breast cancer gene (BRCA) research because they were convenient and available, the participant said. As a result, some of the early discussions referred to BRCA-1 as a "Jewish gene." Had there been an equivalent authority group representing the interests of the original Tay-Sachs population, they might have foreseen this problem, the participant speculated. The participant asked whether lessons from the tribal consultation process should be generalized, and if so, how would people participating in research decide which groups they best fit in? What characteristics of a person or group might need additional representation?

Hiratsuka said that when her organization is approached about using existing study samples for another purpose, she always tries to obtain the viewpoint of the appropriate tribal governing authority and the community members. It is important to ask what the study participants' understanding was regarding the purpose and repurpose of their samples. The practice of a governing body pausing to seek community input to help guide their actions is not distinct to tribal governance, Hiratsuka noted. These types of regional consultations are very important, she said.

Even though race is not a biological determinant of poor health, certain groups, including those that are identified as racial groups, do merit special attention, Roberts clarified. The important question, she reiterated, is What is the purpose of the categories being used by researchers? NIH-funded researchers are required to recruit minorities to their studies and to include race in their data analysis. Researchers often use race as a biological category because they believe NIH requires them to do so, Roberts observed, even when race is not relevant to their research aims. Many also believe that they must report their findings by race and try to draw some conclusion about racial differences. NIH should require that researchers, in working to meet its mandate, consider what is meant by race in the context of the study, why race is relevant to the study, and whether, in fact, the risk factor being studied is not race, but racism.

5

Bioethics Research Workforce

Highlights of Key Points Made by Individual Speakers

- Although legal training is very well suited for bioethics scholarship, lawyers are often not eligible for the training opportunities provided by the National Institutes of Health (NIH) Career Development Awards (K awards), with the exception of a few institutes. (Wilfond)
- The number of individuals receiving NIH K awards for bioethics research is not easy to measure because bioethics is not its own research, condition, and disease category, and, as such, one cannot search the NIH database of scientific awards for the number of bioethics K awards. (Wilfond)
- Bioethics training programs tend to have a topical emphasis (e.g., genomics, neuroethics, palliative care), which results in a lack of opportunities in other areas. (Wilfond)
- In-depth training is needed to be able to produce knowledge on bioethics in low- and middle-income countries. In Latin America and the Caribbean, trainees need to develop the analytic skills required to produce conceptual work. There is also a lack of researchers trained as experts in bioethics in the region. (Saenz)
- Young students interested in the sciences are often also interested in the ethical implications of science, but it is not clear to

them that bioethics itself is a career pathway. There is a need for increased exposure to bioethics training earlier on in the pipeline in order to attract a more diverse group of people to the field of bioethics at an earlier age. (Kahn, Saenz, Wilfond).

- Assessment of workforce development programs, such as the Meyerhoff Scholars Program, is critical to being able to quantitatively demonstrate the impact of the program to financial supporters. (Summers)

- The Meyerhoff approach to increasing interest and involvement in research fields is to expose students to the opportunities for them in these fields, not only as bench scientists, but as leaders. Successful replication of the Meyerhoff Scholars Program model at other institutions is the result of support from upper administration and faculty leadership in making these programs a priority and of inter-institutional partnerships. (Summers)

In this session, panelists discussed the challenges and opportunities associated with conducting bioethics research, including bioethics workforce training and ensuring diversity in the workforce. A U.S. national perspective was provided by Benjamin Wilfond, the director of the Treuman Katz Center for Pediatric Bioethics at Seattle Children's Hospital and Research Institute and a professor in and the chief of the Division of Bioethics and Palliative Care in the Department of Pediatrics at the University of Washington School of Medicine. Carla Saenz, the regional advisor on bioethics at the Pan American Health Organization (PAHO) discussed the conduct of bioethics research from an international perspective. Michael Summers, a professor of chemistry and an investigator with the Howard Hughes Medical Institute (HHMI) at the University of Maryland, Baltimore County (UMBC), described the Meyerhoff Scholars Program as an example of a successful effort to increase diversity in science, technology, engineering, and mathematics (STEM) and related fields. The session was moderated by Maria Merritt of the Johns Hopkins Berman Institute of Bioethics and the Bloomberg School of Public Health.

BIOETHICS TRAINING: A U.S. NATIONAL PERSPECTIVE

Wilfond provided a national view of bioethics training from his perspective as the past president of the Association of Bioethics Program Directors (ABPD) and the chair of the ABPD Funding and Scholarship

Task Force. He also gave his perspectives on bioethics training opportunities through the lens of his role as a co-leader on a multidisciplinary study that includes bioethics research sponsored by the National Human Genome Research Institute (NHGRI).

Current Bioethics Research Training Opportunities

In 1987, when he was a pediatric resident looking for opportunities for bioethics training, there were no formal training programs in bioethics, Wilfond said. Three decades later there are now established bioethics training opportunities for postdoctoral fellows and early- and mid-career scientists, and he shared examples for each career level.

- **Postdoctoral fellows:** Bioethics training available at the postdoctoral level includes individual projects funded by institutional research training grants (NIH T32) or individual postdoctoral fellowships (NIH F32) and established bioethics fellowship programs at institutions across the country (the ABPD website currently lists 17 programs).[1]
- **Early-career faculty:** Training available to early-career research faculty includes the National Institutes of Health (NIH) Career Development Awards (K awards). The number of individuals receiving this training is unknown because bioethics is not an NIH research, condition, and disease (RCD) category, Wilfond said, and as such, one cannot search the NIH database of scientific awards for the number of bioethics K awards. He noted that other types of research, such as data science, are RCD categories, and it would be helpful if bioethics were a searchable category.
- **Mid-career faculty:** Opportunities for mid-career research faculty include The Greenwall Foundation Faculty Scholars Program.[2] A unique and valuable aspect of this program, which has trained 56 scholars since 2003, is that all current and former scholars gather twice each year for ongoing training in support of bioethics scholarship, Wilfond said.

Challenges

Wilfond listed several challenges for bioethics training. First, he said, NIH training programs tend to have a topical emphasis on genomics or

---

[1]See https://www.bioethicsdirectors.net/graduate-bioethics-education-programs-results (accessed April 15, 2020).

[2]See https://greenwall.org (accessed April 15, 2020).

neuroethics. Foundations have focused a lot on palliative care, and this results in a lack of opportunities in other areas. Another concern is that lawyers are not eligible for most NIH K awards, with only a few institutes including them. Wilfond said that those with legal training are perhaps the best suited for bioethics scholarship, and he advocated for this to be changed. Finally, as already noted, it is difficult to identify NIH K award recipients due to the lack of a bioethics RCD category.

Demographics

In preparation for the workshop, ABPD surveyed its members to get a snapshot of the pipeline of people in training for bioethics research careers. Twenty-five of the 70 programs responded, identifying 41 trainees. The majority of the trainees were Ph.D.s (28). The rest had M.D. (7), J.D. (3), or Ph.D./J.D. (2) degrees. Trainees were focused on research ethics (18), clinical ethics (13), or a combination of both (9), Wilfond reported. Ten of the trainees were funded by NIH, but the majority were funded by institutions (25) or other sources (6). Trainees were predominantly female (29) and white (31), and Wilfond said there is a lot of opportunity for increasing the diversity of the trainees. Other trainees identified as Hispanic/Latinx (3), Asian (3), black or African American (2), American Indian or Alaska Native (1), or Native Hawaiian or other Pacific Islander (1).

A Model for Developing Bioethics Research Objectives

The approaches to bioethics research are diverse, Wilfond said, and he briefly described a model for developing bioethics research objectives that was developed by ABPD (Mathews et al., 2016). Together, the type of question (descriptive or prescriptive) and the stage of the question (hypothesis generating or hypothesis testing) drive the selection of the appropriate methodology or approach (see Figure 5-1). Methods can be conceptual or empirical (qualitative or quantitative) or involve consensus/engagement. Wilfond noted that the stages and methods are iterative and that there can be more than one method for a particular type and stage of question.

Incorporating Bioethics Training into Multidisciplinary Studies

In closing, Wilfond said that one opportunity for improving training in bioethics is to take advantage of existing studies. He mentioned one ongoing multidisciplinary study as an example and said that five individuals were able to fund bioethics training through individual awards and supplements (two NIH K Awards that built off the main study, a sexual minority supplement, a diversity supplement, and an administrative supplement).

Question Type →	Descriptive		Prescriptive	
Method				
Conceptual				X
Empirical				
Qualitative		X		
Quantitative	X			
Consensus/Engagement			X	
Question Stage →	Hypothesis generating	Hypothesis testing	Hypothesis generating	Hypothesis testing

FIGURE 5-1 A model for developing bioethics research objectives.
SOURCES: Benjamin Wilfond workshop presentation, February 26, 2020. Concept is originally from Mathews et al. (2016).

Multidisciplinary studies that include bioethics as well as other disciplines represent an opportunity to improve training in bioethics, he said.

BIOETHICS TRAINING IN LATIN AMERICA AND THE CARIBBEAN

An international perspective was provided by Saenz, who focused her remarks on achievements and challenges in bioethics training in Latin America and the Caribbean. In 2014 Saenz and colleagues published an assessment of four bioethics training programs in Latin America and the Caribbean that had been funded by NIH's Fogarty International Center over a 12-year period (Saenz et al., 2014). Conducting this type of study was difficult, Saenz said, because some of the information needed to be obtained directly from the people who were leading the training programs. Program leaders are eager to highlight the accomplishments of their program, and it can be difficult to discuss where the programs are not succeeding, she said.

The conclusion of the assessment, she said, was that the field of research ethics and bioethics training had advanced significantly in the region since 2000, but that some challenges remained. The main challenge identified in all of the training programs in the region, she said, was the need for trainees to develop the analytic skills required to produce conceptual work. The assessment found that the majority of the bioethics research conducted by those who had been trained was descriptive. In preparing for this workshop, Saenz said, she looked back to see how the field had changed in the 6 years since that assessment. She came to the same general conclusion that progress has been made, but some of the same challenges persist.

A subsequent, comprehensive assessment was done of the Fogarty-funded programs across low- and middle-income countries (LMICs) to identify lessons learned and training needs. The main finding, Saenz said, was that individuals require in-depth training to be able to produce knowledge on bioethics. She said this conclusion is particularly relevant to Latin America and the Caribbean. To illustrate, she said if one were to look at articles published in the last 5 or 10 issues of the journal *Developing World Bioethics*, one would find that far fewer articles come from Latin America and the Caribbean than from Africa or Asia, for example.

Advancing Bioethics Training to the Next Level

Bioethics training can be divided into three levels, Saenz said. Level one is very basic training, she said, such as the type of training needed by someone participating on an institutional review board. Level two would be training that might lead to a master's degree in bioethics, for example, and level three would be training researchers to be experts in bioethics. Training programs in Latin America and the Caribbean need to take that last step and develop a cadre of experts for the region, she said. It is not uncommon in Latin America and the Caribbean that those who have taken courses on bioethics at a master's level are expected to teach bioethics. She observed that this does not happen in other disciplines. For example, it is not expected that someone who took a statistics course as part of his or her graduate education would be able to start a biostatistics training program or lead biostatistics research. Bioethics needs to be considered on par with other academic disciplines, Saenz said.

There are three main barriers preventing Latin America and the Caribbean from taking that last step toward increasing regional bioethics expertise, Saenz said. First, she said, it is difficult to train people to develop the practical skills needed for bioethics expertise. It is easier to pass on knowledge than practical skills. There are only a handful of experts in Latin America and the Caribbean, and they are already busy with numerous global projects, she said, and training people is time consuming.

The second barrier, she said, is that "it is very hard to teach new tricks to old dogs." A priority in establishing the bioethics training enterprise was to institutionalize bioethics, Saenz said, but targeting training efforts to mid-career researchers has not led to institutional change. For example, she said, an anesthesiologist who attends a weekly bioethics class will continue being an anesthesiologist and is unlikely to embark on the project of producing knowledge on bioethics. She emphasized the need to start training in bioethics research much earlier in people's careers.

Finally, Saenz said, bioethicists in Latin America and the Caribbean speak a different bioethics "language." For example, she said, cardiologists in Latin America and the Caribbean consume international cardiology literature, engage in a global dialogue, and produce global cardiology knowledge. In contrast, she said, there is limited consumption of international bioethics literature by the bioethicists in the region and also limited production of bioethics literature that meets international standards. Bioethicists need to break out of this cycle and engage in global dialogue on issues that affect the region, she said.

In conclusion, Saenz said that progress is being made through conducting honest, critical assessments of bioethics training programs and collaborating to move programs from level two to level three and increase the bioethics expertise in the countries of the region.

LEARNING FROM WORKFORCE DEVELOPMENT IN SCIENCE, TECHNOLOGY, ENGINEERING, AND MATHEMATICS

Summers described the Meyerhoff Scholars Program at UMBC as a model for creating institutional culture change.[3] The Meyerhoff Scholars Program was started by UMBC president Freeman Hrabowski. As background, Summers said that Hrabowski, who is African American, first came to UMBC in 1987 at a time when black students were protesting because they perceived the campus as racist. Today UMBC leads the country in graduating black M.D.–Ph.D.s, is second in the country in graduating black Ph.D.s (behind Howard University), and is considered a national model for inclusive excellence in STEM, Summers said.

The program was launched in 1989 with 19 male African American students. The program was opened to female African American students in 1990, and in 1996 the program opened to students of all backgrounds who have an interest in the advancement of minorities in STEM fields. Historically, Summers said, about 71 percent of the scholars are underrepresented minorities, about 15 percent are white, and about 14 percent are Asian. Critical support for the program comes from NIH, HHMI, and private donors.

The student-centered program involves cohort learning and immersion in research and attracts high achievers, Summers said. He described the program as "intrusive," with high exposure of the students to research in the learning environment and high expectations for performance. To date there have been approximately 1,500 Meyerhoff participants. Of the more than 1,100 graduates thus far, 91 percent obtained a degree in a STEM field, and 930 graduates have pursued graduate or professional degrees (312 Ph.D.s awarded, 82 percent to minorities; 59 M.D.–Ph.D.s awarded, 90 percent to minorities; 265 STEM master's degrees awarded, 86 percent to minorities; with 258 students currently enrolled in graduate schools, 81 percent of which are minorities).

Program Assessment and Replication

Assessment is critical to be able to quantitatively demonstrate the impact of the program to financial supporters, Summers said. He shared the results of two studies comparing outcomes for Meyerhoff scholars with those of students who declined an offer of admission from the program. Students who enrolled elsewhere graduated with similar grade point averages (GPAs), he said, but were half as likely to graduate with a degree in a STEM field and seven times less likely to obtain a graduate degree in a STEM field (Maton et al., 2009, 2012).

---

[3]For more information, see https://meyerhoff.umbc.edu (accessed April 15, 2020).

The program has also had a broad impact across UMBC. By 2005 there was a 400 percent increase in non-Meyerhoff African American STEM degrees awarded, Summers said. On average, the GPAs of African American students at graduation equaled that of white students, and Meyerhoff program components had been implemented in the broader curriculum, he added. In 2018 the graduation rates for African American students were equal to or exceeded those for white students across all majors.

Beyond UMBC, Summers pointed out that the U.S. Surgeon General Jerome Adams and the principal deputy assistant secretary for health Sylvia Trent-Adams are Meyerhoff Scholars Program alumni. In addition, 40 Meyerhoff alumni hold tenured or tenure-track faculty positions, including positions at Duke University, Stanford University, Johns Hopkins University, and other research universities. Other alumni have chosen to teach at smaller colleges to give back to their communities, he said.

The Meyerhoff Scholars Program, with support from HHMI, partnered with the University of North Carolina at Chapel Hill and The Pennsylvania State University to replicate the program on their campuses. Summers noted that these schools have very different environments and minority compositions, and yet, he said, after 1 year their programs were outperforming the Meyerhoff program, and after 2 years each had raised substantial funding for their endowments (Sto Domingo et al., 2019). This shows that Meyerhoff-like outcomes can rapidly be achieved at large, predominantly majority research universities, Summers said, and he attributed the success to support from like-minded administrative and faculty leadership and inter-institutional partnerships. The Chan Zuckerberg Initiative is currently partnering with UMBC to replicate the Meyerhoff program at the University of California, Berkeley, and the University of California, San Diego.

DISCUSSION

Fostering an Early Interest in Bioethics

There is a need to attract a more diverse group of people to the field of bioethics at an earlier age, Wilfond said. He suggested that there could be an opportunity to draw students to bioethics through the Meyerhoff Scholars Program. The majority of the Meyerhoff scholars care about social justice and societal issues, Summers said, and they have a strong desire to make an impact in their communities. Many of the Meyerhoff students who have gone on to earn their Ph.D. have then done postdoctoral work in policy, he said, because they see this as a pathway to a position where they can have a greater impact on issues they care about. The Meyerhoff approach to increasing interest and involvement in research fields, Summers said, is to expose students to the opportunities open to them in these fields, not only as bench scientists but as leaders. The program prepares them to confidently pursue those positions, he said, and "to not be sidelined by imposter syndrome." The goal, Summers said, is for these students to assume leadership roles in government and academia so that they are in positions to share their experiences on expert panels and be included in discussions of NIH funding priorities, for example.

When considering early engagement initiatives, Saenz said, an important difference to keep in mind is that everyone is exposed to STEM fields early in life, with formal education beginning in elementary school, while exposure to ethics analysis is limited. Thus, the field of bioethics is starting from a disadvantaged position when seeking to attract students. Wilfond observed that young people who are interested in the sciences are also interested in the ethical implications of science and think of ethics as an aspect of the science. It does not occur to them that bioethics is itself a career pathway. What is needed, as discussed by Summers, is exposure to careers in bioethics. Wilfond said he gives a presentation on bioethics careers to a program for underrepresented minorities in the sciences at his institution each year in the hope that someone will become interested. Kahn also agreed that bioethics training is reaching people too late in their careers. Most of the funding is offered at the postgraduate level, and ideally training should be happening at the undergraduate level, Kahn said.

Leading a bioethics research program does not necessarily mean that one is in a "leadership position," Merritt said, noting that many prominent bioethics researchers would not describe themselves as being in a leadership position. She suggested that, for bioethicists, the pathway to leadership is a somewhat different career path than the research path.

Merritt asked about metrics used by the Meyerhoff Scholars Program and about the tracking of students who obtain leadership positions. Summers said that the program is competitive and specifically selects students based on their stated interest in research and demonstrated leadership potential. One of the metrics is how many enter graduate programs after leaving UMBC.

Mentoring in Bioethics

Wilfond suggested that part of what is needed to move bioethics expertise in Latin America and the Caribbean from level two to level three is mentorship. Many of the Fogarty programs include mentorship and collaboration, he said. He asked Saenz what would help the region to create opportunities for bioethicists to advance to that third level of expertise. There is no equivalent of the U.S. style of mentorship in the Latin American and the Caribbean educational systems, Saenz said, noting that professors are paid per hour of instruction. There is no protected time to prepare for and conduct mentoring meetings with students. She added that the majority of research training programs funded by Fogarty in Latin America and the Caribbean involve researchers traveling to a site for a couple of weeks or months and then returning to their regular full-time jobs. In practice, she said, there is little time for continuous mentorship. Because it is unlikely that the system will be redesigned, Saenz suggested that more visiting fellowships could help to fill the mentorship gap for bioethics researchers in Latin America and the Caribbean. In addition, existing fellowships should host more researchers who are at the stage of their careers where they need mentorship to move from level two to level three. In response to a question from Summers, Saenz said that a key advantage of researchers coming together at the international research ethics training programs is immersion. Everyone attending is working in the same area, and part of the learning process is becoming aware of what others are doing as well as getting a "reality check" on what you know and do not know.

Ensuring Diversity Among the Decision Makers

There is a need for greater diversity among those who make the decisions about awarding funding, Merritt said, including the leaders of funding organizations and other sponsors of bioethics research as well institutional boards and university leadership. Summers agreed and said that many programs that began with a focus on increasing the representation of minorities have expanded to include those with socioeconomic differences (e.g., the National Institute of General Medical Sciences Maximizing Access to Research Careers Awards and the Initiative for Maximizing Student Development Program). There are more poor white children in the United States than poor black children, and specific attention is still needed on the issues faced by minority students, Summers said. In the United States, women and minority students are still disadvantaged relative to their white male or Asian male counterparts. Summers reiterated that minority students also suffer from imposter syndrome to a great degree. In addition to calling for more diversity in the leadership of schools and funders, Summers also called for greater racial diversity among NIH research faculty.

Advancing Bioethics Research

Merritt prompted panelists and participants to reflect on what research or actions might be needed to develop greater diversity at every career stage in bioethics. Their suggestions included the following.

Identifying Successful Models of Integrating Bioethics Research into Multidisciplinary Studies

Wilfond briefly described the Cancer Health Assessments Reaching Many (CHARM) study, which is intended to identify interventions that could improve access to genetic testing for diverse populations. The CHARM study involves 10 institutions and 70 people from a wide range of disciplines, including bioethics. One approach to improving bioethics research is to integrate it with other types of research, rather than considering bioethical issues separately, Wilfond said. As such, one area for investigation is identifying and describing successful models of the integration of bioethics research with other disciplines within a project (such as was done for CHARM).

Including the Low- and Middle-Income Country Perspective When Developing Solutions

Saenz reminded participants that LMICs lag behind the United States in institutionalizing basic privacy and research ethics practices. She encouraged participants to include the perspective from LMICs in discussions. Research should not be focused on developing first-world solutions with the expectation that LMICs can just catch up, she said.

Establishing Bioethics Research as a Viable Career Option

Students are savvy when considering career options, Summers said. Areas that are underfunded and do not pay well are not going to draw graduates to postdoctoral fellowship programs. He suggested that to enhance interest among junior researchers, NIH and the National Science Foundation should provide leadership and resources that demonstrate that bioethics is going to be a major area of focus over the next two decades and that funding will be available to early-career investigators.

Filling the Pipeline

Piecing together funding for bioethics training is a concern, Kahn said, but a greater concern is having a pipeline of incoming students to fund. He went on to suggest to Summers that they should discuss how Johns Hopkins University might recruit graduate students from the Meyerhoff Scholars Program.

The pipeline of potential students is increasing as new programs launch, Summers said. There were initially concerns that a Meyerhoff-like program could not succeed at Penn State. Only about 5 percent of students at Penn

State are African American, and it was speculated that the parents of high-achieving black students would be skeptical of the program. Seventy families were invited to the first selection weekend, and 68 families attended. Normally the Meyerhoff Scholars Program at UMBC makes 25 offers of admission because there is funding for 18 students. The program at Penn State made 25 offers and had 23 students accepted, he said, and this trend continues. The key to success is support from upper administration in making these programs a priority, Summers said.

There are a variety of programs helping to fill the pipeline, Summers said. For example, the mayor of Baltimore funds the Baltimore YouthWorks program, which allow Summers to bring about 12 inner-city high school students to work in the laboratories at Johns Hopkins University each summer. The East Baltimore campus of Johns Hopkins University is adjacent to Paul Laurence Dunbar High School, Kahn said, and nearly all of the students there are African American. Faculty from Johns Hopkins are now teaching some of the science curriculum at the high school, and Kahn agreed that the students do not realize that they could someday be doing the same type of work as the researchers who are teaching them. He highlighted the need for approaches to support students entering undergraduate study areas that will prepare them for graduate education and bioethics careers.

Recognizing the Importance of Local Context in Training

It is important to take the local context into account when training the next generation of bioethics researchers, one workshop participant said. Researchers come to the United States for training or to attend training that is provided locally in other parts of the world, but they conduct their research in the context of their own country. Local context shapes the way people operate, how they think about questions, and how they relate those questions to the work they are doing, the participant said, and local context is just as important as training for how they will develop as scholars. It is difficult to "be immersive the other way around" to bring a researcher's context into their training. There is a need to be introspective in considering implicit biases and assumptions about bioethics and to consider how one's views apply in other parts of the world, the participant said. The participant had personally experienced both the benefits of mentorship and training and the challenges of being different, coming into the bioethics research workforce from another discipline and coming to the United States from another country as a person of color.

Commenting on context, Wilfond said that he describes bioethics to nonscientists using three animals of the Pacific Northwest. The salmon swims upstream, and bioethics is similar in many ways, challenging conventional assumptions and asking questions. The penguin is not from the Pacific Northwest, but penguins thrive through collaboration, and collaboration is a critical part of bioethics. The last animal is a 50-foot tall rubber duck in the Tacoma harbor. This rubber duck was originally in Toronto, where it was not simply a rubber duck, but a symbol of U.S. dominance, cultural insensitivity, government excess, and environmental disregard. It is all a matter of perspective, he said, and a fundamental part of bioethics training is to look at things from other perspectives. Collaboration, challenging assumptions, and acknowledging different perspectives are fundamental to bioethics, Wilfond said, regardless of where it is practiced. Several Meyerhoff scholars are from Africa and the Caribbean and they help to bring perspective to discussions of issues such as health care, Summers said.

Funding Doctoral Students' Research in Bioethics

Panelists were asked to comment on whether there should be more support from NIH[4] or other funders for graduate students who want to conduct their doctoral research on bioethics. Saenz fully supported funding more doctoral research and said it would be the easiest way to move from level two of bioethics expertise to level three. Each NIH institute has different mechanisms for supporting people, Wilfond said, and it was discussed among the panel that the NIH F31 award is for predoctoral students. The National Institute of General Medical Sciences has several programs at the undergraduate and graduate levels geared toward increasing diversity, Summers noted. Funding opportunities are very effective in engaging researchers, Wilfond said, noting that the more funding opportunities there are, the more they will be used, making those opportunities important.

Training Research Ethicists for Transdisciplinary Research

A workshop participant observed that embedding ethicists in research projects is an approach that has been taken successfully in the fields of synthetic biology and neuroscience. This requires skills in collaboration and transdisciplinary research in addition to skills in ethics and bioethics, the participant said, going on to ask the panelists how researchers might be trained to fill these types of roles. There is a distinction between an integrated model and an embedded model, Wilfond said. In an integrated model, such as the CHARM study, bioethics is integrated throughout the

---

[4]The Fogarty International Center and NHGRI are part of a bioethics funding opportunity aimed at graduate students, International Bioethics Research Training Program (D43 Clinical Trial Optional). More information on this funding opportunity is available at https://grants.nih.gov/grants/guide/pa-files/PAR-19-243.html (accessed April 29, 2020).

design and conduct of the project. In contrast, an embedded ethicist is readily available to consult as needed.

Saenz said that much of the work she performs at PAHO is the integration of ethics in all of the organization's programs.[5] Ethics is part of the package that PAHO delivers to the member countries it works with, she said. Embedding ethics into these programs requires a high level of expertise in biomedical ethics as well as public health ethics. She pointed out that public health ethics had not been addressed by the workshop, and said that in-depth expertise on ethics should include public health ethics.

The population of older adults is expected to increase significantly in the next 10–15 years, according to a workshop participant. Eighty percent of that population will be living in an LMIC, and one in five will have a mental health condition, the participant continued. Funders such as Fogarty create programs that embed teaching about bioethics into the management of current real-life health issues. For example, digital health will be a critical solution for older adults struggling with mental illness, and perhaps bioethics training could be embedded into the support of these programs, the participant suggested. This is happening to some extent in certain regions, Saenz said, noting that an advantage of this approach is that it gets straight to the discussion and analysis of the issues. A problem with bioethics training in Latin America, Saenz said, is that it is very focused on memorizing, and there is limited attention to deeper ethical analysis. While embedding ethics training into real-life situations provides opportunities for ethics analysis, it does not solve the problem of taking that final step to develop higher-level bioethics expertise.

Clarifying That Normative Research Is Fundable by the National Institutes of Health

A workshop participant recalled the discussion by Saenz that many bioethicists focus on descriptive work and not normative theoretical work,[6] noting that this has also been a critique of NIH-funded ethical, legal, and social implications (ELSI) research. There is a perception among those who receive funding for ELSI research that NIH is less likely to fund normative research and that it favors empirical projects, the participant said. One potential solution would be for NIH requests for applications to state explicitly that normative research is fundable. This finding of the

---

[5] For an overview of the bioethics-related work being conducted by PAHO, see https://www.paho.org/hq/dmdocuments/2013/CSP28-14-e.pdf (accessed April 28, 2020) and https://iris.paho.org/bitstream/handle/10665.2/49706/CD56-INF-21-e.pdf?sequence=1&isAllowed=y (accessed April 28, 2020).

[6] Normative theoretical ethical studies primarily focus on the criteria of what is morally right or wrong, and examine the process by which moral standards are developed.

Fogarty study was somewhat unexpected, Saenz said. The bioethics training program directors are generally more interested in—and are experts on—normative components, but nearly all the trainees produced empirical descriptive bioethics research. This could be because the empirical approach is closer to their background in scientific research, Saenz said.

Normative research is fundable, Wilfond said, who was also aware of the general perception that it is not. He said he often uses a strategy of proposing complementary projects that have both an empirical aim and a normative aim because review groups often have a more difficult time reviewing proposals for conceptual work. ABPD has been involved in communicating to bioethicists that NIH wants to support them and has facilitated NIH giving presentations at bioethics meetings to promote the image of the agency as approachable, Wilfond said.

6

Reflecting on the Workshop and Looking to the Future

In the final session of the workshop, panelists who are potential funders of bioethics research both nationally and internationally reflected on and reacted to the workshop presentations and discussions. Panelists included Tania Simoncelli, the director of policy for science at the Chan Zuckerberg Initiative; Dan O'Connor, the head of humanities and social science at Wellcome Trust; and David Castle, an executive-in-residence at Genome Canada and a professor of public administration at the University of Victoria in British Columbia. The session was moderated by Jeffrey Kahn of Johns Hopkins University, who then called on participants to share their final observations. The rapporteurs' summary of the research topics and areas for further attention that were suggested by individual participants throughout the workshop is included in Box 6-1.

EVOLVING TECHNOLOGIES, RESEARCH MODELS, AND COLLABORATIONS

Ethically Leveraging Digital Technology and Machine Learning for Health

From the information presented, it is clear that the use of digital health technologies, artificial intelligence (AI), and machine learning in biomedical research and clinical care are placing enormous pressure on current privacy, ethics, and regulatory frameworks, Simoncelli said, and one theme that emerged from the workshop was an urgent call for a new system of data sharing and governance. As discussed by Michelle Mello of Stanford University earlier in the day, the ethical issues can be grouped into two main

BOX 6-1
Possible Research Topics and Other Areas
for Further Attention Suggested by
Individual Participants Throughout the Workshop

Over the course of the workshop individual participants suggested a broad range of ideas for further attention and potential funding support in the areas of bioethics, digital technologies, data collection and use, citizen science, structural inequalities around who participates in research, and the workforce training infrastructure for bioethicists and others working in the biomedical fields.

Research Topics

Participants were interested in the following:
- Assessing patients' understanding of their options regarding data sharing, identifying effective approaches for informing them of their options, and determining if educating patients about their options changes their behavior. (Estrin, Mello, Saria, Wilfond)
- Developing and assessing approaches to improving stakeholder literacy about research, data, technology, data management, and ethics. (Estrin, Mello, Nebeker, Ossorio)
- Developing metrics to assess algorithms for bias and fairness. (Ossorio, Saria)
- Evaluating the impact of regulations on ensuring ethical outcomes associated with the use of digital technologies. (Estrin)
- Studying alternative approaches to individual informed consent. (Mello)
- Understanding intergenerational shifts in attitudes toward privacy. (Mello)
- Developing and evaluating different systems of governance and oversight that could be applied to both citizen science and mobile health. (Castle, Merritt, Simoncelli, Wilfond)
- Understanding the health impacts of potential solutions to structural inequities. (Roberts)
- Identifying successful models of integrating bioethics research into multidisciplinary studies. (Wilfond)
- Developing solutions that take into account the perspectives and capabilities of low- and middle-income countries (LMICs) (which can lag behind the United States in institutionalizing basic privacy and research ethics practices). (Saenz)

Other Areas for Attention

Participants discussed the following:
- Engaging researchers in bioethics training earlier in their careers. (Kahn, Saenz, Wilfond)

- Establishing bioethics research as a viable career option for junior researchers, with demonstrated support and leadership from the National Institutes of Health (NIH) and the National Science Foundation. (Summers)
- Increasing the opportunities for mentorship of bioethics researchers, especially researchers from LMICs. (Saenz, Wilfond)
- Preparing undergraduate and graduate students for careers in bioethics, including funding doctoral research on bioethics. (Fabi, Kahn, Saenz, Summers, Wilfond)
- Developing new collaborations across disciplines, institutions, and stakeholders for the ethical development and use of new digital technologies. (Mello, Ossorio, Simoncelli)
- Clarifying that normative research is fundable by NIH. (Ossorio, Saenz, Wilfond)
- Clarifying the application of the Common Rule to research supported by indirect funding. (Wilbanks)
- Mapping out an oversight framework for emerging digital health technologies and related ethical and privacy issues, where funders could play a role by supporting the research that would lay the groundwork for such a framework. (Simoncelli)
- Finding ways to educate, support, and collaborate with citizen and self-researchers to help make their efforts more efficient and ethical (e.g., sharing best practice methods, enabling open science, creating new NIH study sections and quality checklists, funding studies about unregulated research). (Hekler, Simoncelli, Wilbanks)
- Developing a strategic vision for what bioethics encompasses and how it fits into the future of the biomedical research enterprise so that a compelling case for increased funding for bioethics can be made. (O'Connor)
- Redefining what information about an individual's life or health can be reasonably expected to be private in the current technological environment. (Castle, O'Connor)
- Reinforcing the existing principles of bioethics and developing new institutional processes and practices of bioethics that are meaningful and relevant in the current biomedical research ecosystem. (Nebeker, Wilbanks)
- Training those who work in data-intensive sciences and the associated support staff on their roles in the ethical management of data, including safeguarding data privacy. (Castle)
- Creating safe harbors for data-hosting platforms. (Wilbanks)
- Raising researcher awareness of and attention to the worldview of study populations and to the impact of structural inequities on health and disease by engaging with community participants, sociologists, and others who understand structural inequality in society. (Hiratsuka, Roberts)
- Considering what is meant by race in the context of a clinical study and whether and how race as a category is relevant to the study (i.e., is the risk factor under study actually associated with structural inequities). (Roberts)

categories, existing issues compounded by emerging digital technologies and new issues. The reuse of data for purposes that were not originally intended or anticipated is an old problem, for example, but the reuse of data generated by digital technologies brings fresh concerns. An example of a new problem is what Mello termed "the end of anonymity," Simoncelli recounted, where the de-identification of data is no longer sufficient to protect patient privacy. New laws and a new system architecture addressing these issues are needed, she said, and developing them will be extremely challenging. If embedding bioethics into these issues from the start is a priority, as Pilar Ossorio of the University of Wisconsin and others suggested, then perhaps people in the field are already behind, Simoncelli said. As noted by John Wilbanks of Sage Bionetworks, these issues are not likely to be a priority for Congress in the near future. In the interim, Simoncelli said, there is an opportunity to begin mapping out an oversight framework, and perhaps one area where funders could play a role would be to help fund the research that would lay the groundwork for such a framework.

New Collaborations Across Disciplines, Institutions, and Stakeholders

Simoncelli noted that another key theme that had surfaced throughout the day is that one challenge to developing new rules, standards, and solutions to address the ethics issues surrounding the use of digital technologies, AI, and machine learning in health is that none of the stakeholders involved has the full complement of expertise required. For example, she said, regulators are just starting to gain experience with these new technologies that continue to evolve at a rapid pace, and digital technology developers are not trained in ethics. As pointed out earlier in the day by Mello and Ossorio, simply broadening the circle of trust to include digital health technology developers is not the solution because these companies operate under a very different set of norms from those embraced by the clinical research enterprise. This diversity of stakeholder expertise presents an important opportunity for new kinds of collaborations that are multidisciplinary and multi-institutional, Simoncelli said. Although one approach is for stakeholders to bring missing expertise on board (e.g., a technology developer could hire a bioethicist), the discussions advocated for the development of new collaborative spaces where people can come together and "learn each other's language." As an example, Simoncelli said that the Chan Zuckerberg Initiative is a new kind of philanthropy that seeks to address complex challenges by bringing together scientists, engineers, data scientists, policy experts, and advocates.

Incorporating New Models of Research

Another challenge identified for existing regulatory and ethical frameworks is the emergence of alternative approaches to data collection, including citizen science and personal science. As discussed earlier by Eric Hekler of the University of California, San Diego, there is a wide spectrum of ways in which individuals are taking a scientific approach to answering their own questions about their own health and well-being (see Chapter 3). There are many interesting models of community or participant-driven and patient-driven research projects, Simoncelli said, and members of the public are undertaking these efforts because of gaps—both real and perceived—in research that have left the needs of the community unmet. She observed that communities are demanding a more inclusive approach to research and more accountability from the scientific research community. This is another area of great opportunity, Simoncelli said. Patient-driven or patient-partnered research initiatives can benefit research by providing patient insights into their disease areas. Public engagement in science broadly can lead to more support for science. Co-development with communities can lead to new knowledge that is more relevant to the interests and needs of the communities.

At the same time, patients and patient communities are taking on more and more of the burden as they broaden their roles and responsibilities in the research enterprise, Simoncelli said. A question that needs to be asked is whether that is a burden they should have to take on and, if so, how the professional research enterprise might support their efforts. Hiratsuka discussed the role of community leaders in defining the research questions to be asked, the principles of respect and reciprocity that must be adhered to when asking research questions, and what benefit and harm mean in the context of their community. This role of the community is important, but, as Hekler said, it can be somewhat uncomfortable for the professional research community to adapt to the new role of being present but not engaging as they are used to, Simoncelli said. Although there are many new models of citizen and personal research, they are not well studied. Further study is needed to understand which of these new models are most effective and how the research enterprise can best collaborate using them.

VISION AND SCOPE OF BIOETHICS

Making the Business Case for Bioethics

Underlying many of the issues discussed throughout the workshop is the idea that the National Institutes of Health (NIH) needs to spend more money on bioethics, O'Connor said. There are only so many ways to redistribute funds, he said, and more money needs to be dedicated to bioethics. From his perspective as a funder, he said, presenting a compelling vision of what the world will look like—how it will be improved—after the money is spent can influence a funder to support a grant, even when resources are tight.

In this regard O'Connor suggested that NIH needs to develop a vision for how bioethics fits into the future of the biomedical research enterprise. The bioethics community and its collaborators in other fields need to come together and craft a compelling vision of why the world would be better if more money were spent on bioethics. For example, as speakers raised during the workshop, the science will be better if the public is involved, if it is more diverse, and if it addresses and attempts to overcome historical injustices. O'Connor said that bioethics needs to acknowledge the issue of "redistribution of wealth" (i.e., equitable benefit from research). He recalled the discussion by Roberts of gene editing as an example of how those conducting the research have little stake in structural change and often benefit from preserving the status quo. Gene editing, he said, would improve their lives from good to better. There is little attention paid to equitable access and addressing structural injustices. Similarly, as discussed, researchers in for-profit technology companies that develop AI and machine learning for health operate under a different set of norms than those in biomedical research.

Bioethics as a Field of Disciplines

"Bioethics is not a discipline," O'Connor said, "it is a field of many disciplines." Discussions of bioethics are often limited to clinical bioethics. O'Connor observed that "bioethics," as a term, was used broadly throughout the workshop. Disciplines in the field of bioethics often include law, philosophy, and clinical research. Based on the scope of the workshop discussions, he suggested that the disciplines of sociology, the history of medicine, critical medical humanities, science and technology studies, and literary theory are also necessary.

Bioethics as a field includes disciplines that NIH has classically not funded, and O'Connor highlighted the need to look at the structures of grant making and ensure that the decision makers are diverse and have the disciplinary backgrounds needed to meet the interdisciplinary challenges of bioethics. Panelists discussed diversity as it relates to bioethics research and the training of the bioethics workforce. In the past, he said, the vision put forth by the bioethics community was essentially that all research would be conducted ethically. This vision is insufficient to encompass the expansive scope of what is meant by "bioethics" as used throughout the workshop. O'Connor highlighted the need for a broader strategic vision for what bioethics will be. This vision should define the standards for what is ethical and make judgments accordingly, and it should demonstrate that bioethics can be both the study of and the enabler of science, he said.

Castle expanded the discussion of the disciplinary status of bioethics, sharing his perspective on how considering bioethics to be a discipline can be a problem. To illustrate, he described the Genomics and its Ethical, Environmental, Economic, Legal and Social Aspects (GE[3]LS) program of Genome Canada.[1] The program is similar to the ethical, legal, and social implications program in the United States and to the ethical, legal, and social aspects programs in Europe. The scope of GE[3]LS includes biomedical, environmental, agricultural, social sciences and humanities, and legal scholarship. Castle said that social sciences and humanities research tended to be part of the large-scale applied research programs and that it is mandated by Genome Canada that there be an integrated social sciences and humanities research component built in. One challenge for these projects, he said, has been to form interdisciplinary teams in which there is genuine interaction between the natural and social sciences. Another challenge is to sustain interdisciplinary research interactions and to be able to distinguish the research outputs from having large-scale, integrated programs that deliver socioeconomic benefits.

A benefit of Genome Canada's integrative approach, Castle said, is that GE[3]LS provides a new funding stream for social sciences and humanities researchers for both conceptual and applied research. In some cases, he said, they can see the impact of their work in the real world. A disadvantage of this approach, which Castle suggested is related to the disciplinary status of bioethics, is that it can be difficult to recruit researchers to the projects. One reason is that they might not believe that they have the kind of disciplinary or interdisciplinary focus that is needed, a perspective that may be shaped and entrenched by responding to traditional funding sources. Another reason is that social scientists are used to working with other social scientists and humanities researchers, and the idea of conducting integrated, interdisciplinary work with natural scientists or clinical scientists is challenging, especially for early-career researchers who are trying to establish themselves within the conventions of their particular disciplines.

DISCUSSION

Taking on the Burdens of Self Science

There is a collective action problem among citizens and patients, suggested Maria Merritt of Johns Hopkins University. She recalled the debate about whether individuals should be accepting free services from a digi-

---

[1]For more information, see https://www.genomecanada.ca/en/programs/genomics-society-ge3ls (accessed April 15, 2020).

tal platform in exchange for access to their data and the point made by Simoncelli that patients are bearing more and more of the burden that really should not be theirs to bear. There is not an organized way in which individuals can protect their own interests or articulate them collectively, Merritt said. With respect to the concerns raised about not being able to regulate these emerging technologies within the existing system, she pointed out that the European Union has a very different regulatory regime from the United States, and she suggested it might be worth comparing the approaches to governance.

Castle said that this is a key action area for intellectual inquiry and for funding. There is enough evidence available on how big data is being handled and on how corporate interests retain the autonomy to self-regulate to take action. He suggested that the time to reform or regulate these issues has passed and that what is needed is a fundamental re-orientation to a changed world. He acknowledged the concerns about the sale and reuse of data but added that "a fortress mentality" around health data can actually stifle innovation. As an example, he said that where he lives in Canada, the previous privacy commissioner publicly admonished the Ministry of Health twice, claiming that they were keeping useful data out of the hands of innovators and preventing possible research and development partnerships that could help the population. Issuing this type of warning is very unusual for them, Castle said, because the unelected officials in the ministry were overly risk averse.

Simoncelli elaborated on the increasing burden on patient communities. There are many contexts and ways in which patients are seeking access to their data, she said. For example, although patients have the right to their health records under the Health Insurance Portability and Accountability Act, one's data are not necessarily easy to obtain. Another area where patients are taking on an increasing burden is rare disease research. More and more, rare disease communities are building the research-enabling infrastructure needed to attract researchers and to accelerate research on rare diseases that have been neglected by traditional academic research. She said that there is no real infrastructure to support this patient-driven model of research; groups are organizing themselves and creating what they need from the ground up. In that regard, she suggested, this approach is part of a broader patient movement focused on accelerating research on the terms of patients, and this movement could bring current bioethical issues to the forefront.

Bioethics for the Benefit of Society

Discussions about broadening the conception of what bioethics is and developing a strategic vision for bioethics are important, a workshop participant said. That vision, she said, is that bioethics is necessary to make society better. She said that she formerly worked at NIH in a funding role, and she added that there was pressure from the leadership of the scientific programs that any funding for bioethics had to be in the context of how bioethics can make scientific research better. As a result, she said, it was difficult to make programmatic decisions to support bioethics work in a more comprehensive way. The justification for work in bioethics is not that it is an adjunct to doing good research. The justification for bioethics is that making society better involves using all of the tools available to improve people's lives, including structural and biomedical tools as well as bioethics and other interdisciplinary tools, she said.

Castle agreed and said that Genome Canada has a fundamental social mission of doing the scientific research and technology development to improve lives and increase prosperity. The challenge, he said, is to create programs that deliver on that mission. Castle said that the organization is updating review criteria and guidance to include examples of what meaningful integration of natural and social sciences looks like. It is not enough to simply add on a bioethicist as an afterthought and call it "interdisciplinary," he said. In addition, the Genome Canada program structure permits the funding of projects that stem from a social sciences and humanities viewpoint. As an example, he mentioned a funded project for which the central question involved using genomics tools to enable remediation in forestry. Development of the project started with a consultation process, led by indigenous communities, to set the priorities from their perspective about what was happening on their lands. The science was then structured around those priorities, resulting in an integrated project with a clear deliverable back to the affected communities, he said.

At Wellcome Trust, O'Connor said, the funding strategy within the humanities and social sciences and the disciplines that make up the broad field of bioethics is to determine what the organization excels at that can add value for finding solutions. For example, Wellcome Trust funds literary studies, which O'Connor said can add to the understanding of how people and communities experience illness. The skills and expertise found in the humanities and the social sciences can help to elucidate the lived experience and form questions in a way that science does not. O'Connor said that the disciplines within the field of bioethics need to confidently offer to contribute their skills and expertise to solutions.

Bioethicists' Role in Rapid Response

Kahn said that one of the ways in which bioethicists are valuable is that they are available to help address emerging ethical issues as they arise (e.g., issues associated with the novel coronavirus outbreak[2]). One barrier to providing a rapid response can be the need to go through investigator-initiated research proposals for support, and Kahn suggested that there is an opportunity to discuss this further. O'Connor said that rapid reaction depends on the availability of people who have the depth of training and broad expertise needed. The challenge for funders is to justify supporting an activity that is not needed all the time, even though it is of high value at those times when it is needed. This is particularly difficult for a public funder, such as NIH, that is accountable to the government and the tax-payers, O'Connor said. As a private foundation, Wellcome Trust has a moral duty to fill the gap and fund these types of activities that its public colleagues cannot. However, Wellcome Trust does not have the scale and scope that NIH does. He suggested that there is an opportunity for NIH to make some funding available to enable the rapid availability of bioethics capacity, and he reiterated that this requires making the case confidently for why this is of value. Wilfond noted that the National Center for Advancing Translational Sciences' Clinical and Translational Science Awards Program originally required institutions to have an ethics component as part of their awards. Although this is no longer a requirement, he said that an element that has been sustained consists of the institutional research ethics consulta-tion services, which he said offer support to investigators who do not have embedded ethicists in their programs.

Redefining What Information Can Reasonably Be Expected to Be Private

The definition of private information as it pertains to human subjects should be considered, said a workshop participant. Per the Common Rule, "private information includes information about behavior that occurs in a context in which an individual can reasonably expect that no observation or recording is taking place."[3] When that definition was originally written, he said, the sense was that people did not have a reasonable expectation that information in publicly available sources was private (e.g., listings in the phone book, court records) or that what they might do out in public would remain private (e.g., researchers observing people in a public space). Today, given the volume of information available on the Internet and the ways in which those data can be combined to develop a picture of a person's life,

---

[2]At the time of the workshop, the U.S. Centers for Disease Control and Prevention had just confirmed the possibility of community spread of COVID-19 in the United States. See https://www.cdc.gov/media/releases/2020/s0226-Covid-19-spread.html (accessed April 20, 2020). On March 11, 2020, the World Health Organization declared COVID-19 a pandemic. See https://www.who.int/dg/speeches/detail/who-director-general-s-opening-remarks-at-the-media-briefing-on-covid-19---11-march-2020 (accessed April 20, 2020).

[3]45 CFR 46.102(e)(4).

the workshop participant asked whether anyone could have the reasonable expectation that any information about their lives or health is private. He suggested there is a need to revisit this definition and what it was originally intended to protect and to consider how it might be refined to protect that interest in the current technological environment. Castle agreed that further discussion is needed on what would be a reasonable expectation of privacy in light of current norms. He suggested that, in addition to legal and ethical analyses, there should also be empirical analysis to understand, for example, the contextualization of data and how thresholds of expectations change as the technological landscape changes. O'Connor added that moral norms and notions of privacy change over time. Some of the disciplines in the field of bioethics, such as anthropology, sociology, and science and technology studies, can help to define current experiences and expectations of privacy, which can inform the discussions of the definition of private information.

Workforce Training Considerations

Castle also highlighted the need for training those who work in data-intensive sciences and the associated support staff on their roles in safeguarding data privacy. A workshop participant agreed that the researchers who are actually using these data (and who do not interact with the patients contributing the data) need training in the ethical management of the data (e.g., data use, combining data). Castle said that there is a wide spectrum of issues that are being incorporated into curricula to help data scientists and those who work with them to be better stewards and users of data. Ethical issues that researchers might face include, for example, structural bias in the data; unintended consequences of algorithm development use; the potential for dual use of algorithms, applying data from one domain to another domain it was not intended for (e.g., applying AI to data for law enforcement purposes); or using data from social media for behavioral modeling that is then used to fundamentally change people's choice architectures.

CLOSING REMARKS

A main theme of the workshop was disruptive shifts in relationships along a number of axes, Kahn said—shifts in the relationship that individuals have with data that are from or about them and with the professionals who use their data; shifts in the notion of how communities and citizens relate to science, and how science relates to communities and citizens; shifts in how researchers ought to be thinking about inequality and research participation and the implications of research; and shifts in the relationship research has with the workforce pipeline in bioethics. All of these disruptive shifts are making the world hopefully better, he concluded, but certainly different.

References

Buolamwini, J., and T. Gebru. 2018. Gender shades: Intersectional accuracy disparities in commercial gender classification. *Proceedings of Machine Learning Research* 81:1–15.

Cohen, I. G., and M. M. Mello. 2019. Big data, big tech, and protecting patient privacy. *JAMA* 322(12):1141–1142.

Coravos, A., I. Chen, A. Gordhandas, and A. D. Stern. 2019. We should treat algorithms like prescription drugs. *Quartz*, February 14. https://qz.com/1540594/treating-algorithms-like-prescription-drugs-could-reduce-ai-bias (accessed April 15, 2020).

Du Bois, W. E. B. 1899. *The Philadelphia Negro*. Philadelphia: University of Pennsylvania Press.

EC (European Commission). 2014. *Green paper on citizen science for Europe: Towards a society of empowered citizens and enhanced research.* https://ec.europa.eu/digital-single-market/en/news/green-paper-citizen-science-europe-towards-society-empowered-citizens-and-enhanced-research (accessed April 15, 2020).

Flier, J. S., and J. Loscalzo. 2017. Categorizing biomedical research: The basics of translation. *FASEB Journal* 31(8):3210–3215. https://doi.org/10.1096/fj.201700303R.

Goodfellow, I. J., J. Shlens, and C. Szegedy. 2015. *Explaining and harnessing adversarial examples.* Conference paper presented at the 2015 International Conference on Learning Representations, San Diego, CA. https://arxiv.org/pdf/1412.6572.pdf (accessed April 15, 2020).

Grant, A. D., G. Wolf, and C. Nebeker. 2019. Approaches to governance of participant-led research: A qualitative case study. *BMJ Open* 9(4):e025633.

Hand, D. 2018. Aspects of data ethics in a changing world: Where are we now? *Big Data* 6(3):176–190.

Heigl, F., B. Kieslinger, K. T. Paul, J. Uhlik, and D. Dörler. 2019. Opinion: Toward an international definition of citizen science. *Proceedings of the National Academy of Sciences* 116(17):8089–8092.

Heyen, N. B. 2020. From self-tracking to self-expertise: The production of self-related knowledge by doing personal science. *Public Understanding of Science* 29(2):124–138.

Kirschenbaum, M.A., M. L. Birnbaum, A. Rizvi, W. Muscat, L. Patel, and J. M. Kane. 2019. Google search activity in early psychosis: A qualitative analysis of internet search query content in first episode psychosis. *Early Intervention in Psychiatry.* https://doi.org/10.1111/eip.12886 [Epub ahead of print].

Kistka, Z. A. F., L. Palomar, K. A. Lee, F. S. Cole, M. R. DeBaun, and L. J. Muglia. 2007. Racial disparity in the frequency of recurrence of preterm birth. *American Journal of Obstetrics and Gynecology* 196(2):131.e1–131.e6.

Mathews, D. J. H., D. M. Hester, J. Kahn, A. McGuire, R. McKinney, K. Meador, S. Philpott-Jones, S. Youngner, and B. S. Wilfond. 2016. A conceptual model for the translation of bioethics research and scholarship. *Hastings Center Report* 46:34–39.

Maton, K. I., M. R. Sto Domingo, K. E. Stolle-McAllister, J. L. Zimmerman, and F. A. Hrabowski 3rd. 2009. Enhancing the number of African Americans who pursue STEM Ph.D.s: Meyerhoff Scholarship Program outcomes, processes, and individual predictors. *Journal of Women and Minorities in Science and Engineering* 15(1):15–37.

Maton, K. I., S. A. Pollard, T. V. McDougall Weise, and F. A. Hrabowski. 2012. Meyerhoff Scholars Program: A strengths-based, institution-wide approach to increasing diversity in science, technology, engineering, and mathematics. *Mount Sinai Journal of Medicine* 79(5):610–623.

Metcalf, J. 2014. *Ethics codes: History, context, and challenges.* Council for Big Data, Ethics, and Society. https://bdes.datasociety.net/council-output/ethics-codes-history-context-and-challenges (accessed April 20, 2020).

Miller, B. 2013. When is consensus knowledge based? Distinguishing shared knowledge from mere agreement. *Synthese* 190(7):1293–1316.

Millum. J., B. Sina, and R. Glass. 2015. International research ethics education. *JAMA* 313(5):461–462.

Nissenbaum, H. 2011. A contextual approach to privacy Online. *Daedalus* 140:32–48.

Nissenbaum, H. 2018. Respecting context to protect privacy: Why meaning matters. *Science and Engineering Ethics* 24(3):831–852.

Obermeyer, Z., B. Powers, C. Vogeli, and S. Mullainathan. 2019. Dissecting racial bias in an algorithm used to manage the health of populations. *Science* 366(6464):447–453.

Price, W. N. 2nd, and I. G. Cohen. 2019. Privacy in the age of medical big data. *Nature Medicine* 25(1):37–43.

Quiñonero-Candela, J., M. Sugiyama, A. Schwaighofer, and N. D. Lawrence. 2009. *Dataset shift in machine learning.* Cambridge, MA: The MIT Press.

Roberts, D. 2018. *Fatal invention: How science, politics and big business recreate race in the 21st Century.* New York: The New Press.

Rothstein, M. A., J. Wilbanks, L. M. Beskow, K.Brelsford, K. Brothers, M. Doerr, B. J. Evans, C. Hammack, M. McGowan, and S. A. Tovino. 2020. Unregulated health research using mobile devices: Ethical considerations and policy recommendations. *Journal of Law, Medicine & Ethics* 48(Suppl 1):196–226.

Saenz, C., E. Heitman, F. Luna, S. Litewka, K. W. Goodman, and R. Macklin. 2014. Twelve years of Fogarty-funded bioethics training in Latin America and the Caribbean: Achievements and challenges. *Journal of Empirical Research on Human Research Ethics* 9(2):80–91.

Saha, K., L. Chan, K. De Barbaro, G. D. Abowd, and M. De Choudhury. 2017. Inferring mood instability on social media by leveraging ecological momentary assessments. *Proceedings of the ACM on Interactive, Mobile, Wearable, and Ubiquitous Technologies* 1(3).

Saria, S., and A. Subbaswamy. 2019. *Tutorial: Safe and reliable machine learning.* Presented at the 2019 Association for Computing Machinery (ACM) Conference on Fairness, Accountability, and Transparency. https://arxiv.org/pdf/1904.07204.pdf (accessed April 15, 2020).

Sharon, T. 2016. The Googlization of health research: From disruptive innovation to disruptive ethics. *Personalized Medicine* 13(6):563–574.

Solove, D. 2020. The myth of the privacy paradox. *GW Law Faculty Publications & Other Works*. No. 1482. https://scholarship.law.gwu.edu/faculty_publications/1482 (accessed April 30, 2020).

Sto Domingo, M. R., S. Sharp, A. Freeman, T. Freeman Jr, K. Harmon, M. Wiggs, V. Sathy, A. T. Panter, L. Oseguera, S. Sun, M. E. Williams, J. Templeton, C. L. Folt, E. J. Barron, F. A. Hrabowski 3rd, K. I. Maton, M. Crimmins, C. R. Fisher, and M. F. Summers. 2019. Replicating Meyerhoff for inclusive excellence in STEM. *Science* 364(6438):335–337.

Subbaswamy, A., and S. Saria. 2020. From development to deployment: Dataset shift, causality, and shift-stable models in health AI. *Biostatistics* 21(2):345–352.

van der Zee, T., and J. Reich. 2018. Open Education Science. *AERA Open* 4(3):1–15.

White, R. W., P. Murali Doraiswamy, and E. Horvitz. 2018. Detecting neurodegenerative disorders from web search signals. *npj Digital Medicine* 1:8.

Wiens, J., S. Saria, M. Sendak, M. Ghassemi, V. Liu, F. Doshi-Velez, K. Jung, K. Heller, D. Kale, M. Saeed, P. N. Ossorio, S. Thadaney-Israni, and A. Goldenberg. 2019. Do no harm: A roadmap for responsible machine learning for health care. *Nature Medicine* 25(9):1337–1340.

Zech, J. R., M. A. Badgeley, M. Liu, A. B. Costa, J. J. Titano, and E. K. Oermann. 2018. Variable generalization performance of a deep learning model to detect pneumonia in chest radiographs: A cross-sectional study. *PLOS Medicine* 15(11):e1002683.

Appendix A

Workshop Agenda

Keck Center of the National Academies
Room 100
500 Fifth Street, NW
Washington, DC 20001

8:30 a.m. **Opening Remarks and Charge to Workshop Speakers and Participants**

JEFFREY KAHN
Andreas C. Dracopoulos Director
Robert Henry Levi and Ryda Hecht Levi Professor of Bioethics and Public Policy
Berman Institute of Bioethics
Professor
Health Policy and Management
Bloomberg School of Public Health
Johns Hopkins University

SESSION I: DEVELOPING, TESTING, AND INTEGRATING NEW DIGITAL TECHNOLOGIES INTO RESEARCH AND CLINICAL CARE

Session Moderator: Bernard Lo, The Greenwall Foundation

8:45 a.m.   DEBORAH ESTRIN
Associate Dean and Robert V. Tishman '37 Professor
Cornell NYC Tech

9:00 a.m.   MICHELLE MELLO
Professor of Law and Medicine
Stanford University

SESSION II: USING ARTIFICIAL INTELLIGENCE AND MACHINE LEARNING IN RESEARCH AND CLINICAL CARE

Session Moderator: Bernard Lo, The Greenwall Foundation

9:15 a.m.   SUCHI SARIA
John C. Malone Assistant Professor
Departments of Computer Science and Health Policy and
Management
Johns Hopkins University

9:30 a.m.   PILAR OSSORIO
Professor of Law and Bioethics
University of Wisconsin

9:45 a.m.   **Panel Discussion with Speakers from Sessions I and II**

10:45 a.m.   **Break**

SESSION III: ETHICAL QUESTIONS AROUND NONTRADITIONAL APPROACHES FOR DATA COLLECTION AND USE

Session Moderator: Camille Nebeker, University of California, San Diego

11:00 a.m.   ERIC HEKLER
             Associate Professor
             Department of Family Medicine and Public Health
             University of California, San Diego

11:15 a.m.   JOHN WILBANKS
             Chief Commons Officer
             Sage Bionetworks

11:30 a.m.   **Panel Discussion with Speakers and Workshop Participants**

             ERIC HEKLER
             JOHN WILBANKS

             CAMILLE NEBEKER
             Associate Professor
             School of Medicine
             University of California, San Diego

12:00 p.m.   **Break for Lunch**

SESSION IV: UNDERSTANDING THE IMPACT OF INEQUALITY ON HEALTH, DISEASE, AND WHO PARTICIPATES IN RESEARCH

Moderator: Anita Allen, University of Pennsylvania

1:15 p.m.   DOROTHY ROBERTS
             George A. Weiss University Professor of Law and Sociology
             Raymond Pace and Sadie Tanner Mossell Alexander
             Professor of Civil Rights
             University of Pennsylvania

1:30 p.m.   VANESSA HIRATSUKA
             Senior Researcher
             Southcentral Foundation

1:45 p.m.   **Panel Discussion with Speakers and Workshop Participants**

SESSION V: CHALLENGES AND OPPORTUNITIES IN THE BIOETHICS RESEARCH WORKFORCE INFRASTRUCTURE AND FOR ENSURING DIVERSITY

Session Moderator: Maria Merritt, Johns Hopkins University

2:15 p.m.   BEN WILFOND
            Director
            Treuman Katz Center for Pediatric Bioethics
            Seattle Children's Hospital and Research Institute
            Professor and Chief
            Division of Bioethics and Palliative Care, Department of
            Pediatrics
            University of Washington School of Medicine

2:20 p.m.   CARLA SAENZ
            Regional Advisor on Bioethics
            Pan American Health Organization

2:25 p.m.   MICHAEL SUMMERS
            Professor of Chemistry and Investigator
            Howard Hughes Medical Institute
            University of Maryland, Baltimore County

2:30 p.m.   **Moderated Discussion with Panelists**

3:00 p.m.   **Questions from Workshop Participants**

3:30 p.m.   **Break**

SESSION VI: LOOKING TO THE FUTURE AND ANTICIPATING ETHICAL ISSUES RELATED TO BIOMEDICAL RESEARCH

SESSION OBJECTIVES:
 • Discuss the action items covered during the day and what is needed
   to prepare for and address the challenges of emerging bioethical
   issues over the next 5–10 years.

Session Moderator: Jeffrey Kahn, Johns Hopkins University

3:45 p.m.   Reactions from Stakeholders

              TANIA SIMONCELLI
              Director of Policy for Science
              Chan Zuckerberg Initiative

              DAN O'CONNOR
              Head of Humanities and Social Science
              Wellcome Trust

              DAVID CASTLE
              Executive-in-Residence
              Genome Canada
              Professor of Public Administration
              University of Victoria

4:00 p.m.   Discussion with Workshop Participants

4:30 p.m.   Insights from the Day's Discussions

              JEFFREY KAHN
              Andreas C. Dracopoulos Director
              Robert Henry Levi and Ryda Hecht Levi Professor of
              Bioethics and Public Policy
              Berman Institute of Bioethics
              Professor
              Health Policy and Management
              Bloomberg School of Public Health
              Johns Hopkins University

4:45 p.m.   Concluding Remarks

5:00 p.m.   Adjourn

Appendix B

Speaker Biographical Sketches

Anita LaFrance Allen, J.D., Ph.D. (NAM), is an internationally renowned expert on privacy law and ethics and is recognized for contributions to legal philosophy, women's rights, and diversity in higher education. In July 2013 Dr. Allen was appointed the University of Pennsylvania vice provost for faculty and in 2015 the chair of the Penn Provost's Advisory Council on Arts, Culture and the Humanities. From 2010 to 2017 she served on President Obama's Presidential Commission for the Study of Bioethical Issues. She was presented the Lifetime Achievement Award of the Electronic Privacy Information Center in 2015 and elected to the National Academy of Medicine in 2016. In 2017 Dr. Allen was elected vice-president/president elect of the Eastern Division of the American Philosophical Association. In 2015 she was on the summer faculty of the School of Criticism and Theory at Cornell University. A 2-year term as an associate of the Johns Hopkins Humanities Center concluded in 2018. Her books include *Unpopular Privacy: What Must We Hide* (Oxford, 2011), *Privacy Law and Society* (Thomson/West, 2017), *The New Ethics: A Guided Tour of the 21st Century Moral Landscape* (Miramax/Hyperion, 2004), and *Why Privacy Isn't Everything: Feminist Reflections on Personal Accountability* (Rowman and Littlefield, 2003).

David Castle, Ph.D., is a professor in the School of Public Administration and the Gustavson School of Business at the University of Victoria (UVic). He recently served as the vice president of research at UVic and was previously the director of the Innogen Institute at the University of Edinburgh. With expertise in science, technology, and innovation policy, his research is focused on large-scale research infrastructure and big science, intellectual property and research data management, and the social determinants of innovation and new technology regulation and adoption. He is the co-author of *Canadian Science, Technology and Innovation Policy: The Innovation Economy and Society Nexus* and of several works on biotechnology innovation, regulation, and intellectual property. An experienced executive leader in postsecondary education, he has consulted widely on governance and strategy, particularly with respect to interactions among government, private, and voluntary sectors.

Deborah Estrin, Ph.D., is a professor of computer science at Cornell NYC Tech, where she founded the Health Tech Hub in the Jacobs Institute and the Small Data Lab at Cornell NYC Tech. She is the Robert V. Tishman '37 Professor and an associate dean. Her current research focus is at the intersection of small data, personalization, and privacy. Much of her prior work focused on leveraging the pervasiveness of mobile devices and digital interactions for health and life management. Dr. Estrin co-founded the nonprofit startup Open mHealth and served on several scientific advisory boards for early-stage mobile health startups. She recently began as a part-time Amazon Scholar. Previously, Dr. Estrin was on the University of California, Los Angeles, faculty where she was the founding director of the National Science Foundation Center for Embedded Networked Sensing, pioneering the development of mobile and wireless systems to collect and analyze real-time data about the physical world. Her honors include the ACM Athena Lecture (2006), Anita Borg Institute's Women of Vision Award for Innovation (2007), the American Academy of Arts & Sciences (2007), the National Academy of Engineering (2009), the IEEE Internet Award (2017), a MacArthur fellow (2018), and, most recently, the National Academy of Medicine (2019).

Eric Hekler, Ph.D., is the director of the Center for Wireless and Population Health Systems within the Qualcomm Institute at the University of California, San Diego (UCSD), an associate professor in the Department of Family Medicine and Public Health, and a member of the faculty of the Design Lab at UCSD. There are three interdependent themes to his research: (1) advancing methods for optimizing adaptive behavioral interventions; (2) advancing methods and processes to help people help themselves, particularly N-of-1 methods; and (3) advancing the research pipelines to equitably improve people's health efficiently. He is internationally recognized as an expert in the area of digital health.

Vanessa Hiratsuka (Diné/Winnemem Wintu), Ph.D., M.P.H., is a public health researcher with more than 19 years of mixed methods research experience within the Alaska tribal health system. She received a bachelor's degree in human biology from Stanford University, a master's degree in public health practice from the University of Alaska Anchorage, and a doctoral degree in public health from Walden University. Her community engagement work has spanned regional, national, and international efforts. She has extensive experience coaching and mentoring community and university-based researchers and practitioners in the ethical, social, and legal implications of genomic research and clinical and translational research in tribal health settings.

Jeffrey Kahn, Ph.D., M.P.H. (NAM), is the Andreas C. Dracopoulos Director of the Johns Hopkins Berman Institute of Bioethics, a position he assumed in July 2016. Since 2011 he has been the inaugural Robert Henry Levi and Ryda Hecht Levi Professor of Bioethics and Public Policy. He is also a professor in the Department of Health Policy and Management of the Johns Hopkins Bloomberg School of Public Health. He works in a variety of areas of bioethics, exploring the intersection of ethics and health/science policy, including human and animal research ethics, public health, and ethical issues in emerging biomedical technologies. Dr. Kahn has served on numerous state and federal advisory panels. He is currently the chair of the National Academies of Sciences, Engineering, and Medicine's Board on Health Sciences Policy, and he previously chaired its Committee on the Use of Chimpanzees in Biomedical and Behavioral Research (2011); the Committee on Ethics Principles and Guidelines for Health Standards for Long Duration and Exploration Spaceflights (2014); and the Committee on the Ethical, Social, and Policy Considerations of Mitochondrial Replacement Techniques (2016). He also formerly served as a member of the National Institutes of Health (NIH) Recombinant DNA Advisory Committee. In addition to his committee leadership and membership, Dr. Kahn is an elected member of the National Academy of Medicine and an elected fellow of The Hastings Center. He was also the founding president of the Association of Bioethics Program Directors, an office he held from 2006 to 2010.

Dr. Kahn is a co-principal investigator with Berman Institute faculty member Gail Geller on GUIDE: Genomic Uses in Infectious Disease and Epidemics, an NIH-funded project to study the largely unexplored ethical, legal, and social implications of genomics as applied to infectious disease. Dr. Kahn's publications include *Contemporary Issues in Bioethics; Beyond Consent: Seeking Justice in Research* and *Ethics of Research with Human Subjects: Selected Policies and Resources* as well as more than 125 scholarly and research articles. He also speaks widely across the United States and around the world on a range of bioethics topics in addition to frequent media outreach. From 1998 to 2002 he wrote the bi-weekly column *Ethics Matters* on CNN.com. Prior to joining the faculty at Johns Hopkins University, Dr. Kahn was the director of the Center for Bioethics at the University of Minnesota.

Cecil Lewis, Ph.D., is a professor at the University of Oklahoma. His research falls under the broad umbrella of molecular anthropology, with a particular focus on population history, human evolution, and what could be described as microbial anthropology. During his tenure at the University of Oklahoma, it has been his objective to foster leadership in research that bridges microbial and anthropological sciences. He has led research featured in several news outlets, including *Science, Discover, National Geographic, New Scientist,* and more. He has published in high-impact journals, including *Nature Genetics, Nature Communications, Proceedings of the National Academy of Sciences, Current Biology, PLOS Genetics,* and others. His research has been supported by the National Science Foundation (including a CAREER award), the National Institutes of Health (including three R01s and a "Center for Excellence" grant), and other agencies.

Bernard Lo, M.D. (NAM), is the president and the chief executive officer of The Greenwall Foundation. Before this, Dr. Lo was a professor of medicine and the director of the Program in Medical Ethics at the University of California, San Francisco. He is the co-chair of the Standards Working Group of the California Institute of Regenerative Medicine. He serves on the board of directors of the Association for the Accreditation of Human Research Protection Programs. A member of the National Academy of Medicine, Dr. Lo served on the Institute of Medicine (IOM) Council, chaired the National Academies' Board on Health Sciences Policy, and chaired an IOM report on conflicts of interest in medicine, research, education, and practice.

Michelle Mello, J.D., Ph.D., M.Phil., is a professor of law at Stanford Law School and a professor of medicine in the Center for Health Policy/ Primary Care and Outcomes Research in the Department of Medicine at the Stanford University School of Medicine. She conducts empirical research into issues at the intersection of law, ethics, and health policy. She is the author of nearly 200 articles and book chapters on medical liability, public health law, pharmaceuticals and vaccines, biomedical research ethics and governance, health information privacy, and other topics. The recipient of a number of awards for her research, Dr. Mello was elected to the National Academy of Medicine at the age of 40. From 2000 to 2014 she was a professor at the Harvard T.H. Chan School of Public Health, where she directed the school's program in law and public health. Dr. Mello holds a J.D. from the Yale Law School and a Ph.D. in health policy and administration from the University of North Carolina at Chapel Hill.

Maria Merritt, Ph.D., is a core faculty member of the Johns Hopkins Berman Institute of Bioethics. A major objective of Dr. Merritt's current research, in collaboration with colleagues, is to develop a novel methodology for considering social justice impacts side-by-side with cost effectiveness as a part of economic evaluation in health policy. Dr. Merritt's other areas of scholarly interest include the ethics of public health research in low- and middle-income countries—particularly questions about researchers' responsibilities to benefit research participants and populations—and moral psychology, the study of feeling, thought, and action in morally significant contexts. Dr. Merritt serves as the associate chair for student matters in the Johns Hopkins Bloomberg School of Public Health Department of International Health and as a program officer for the Johns Hopkins University Exploration of Practical Ethics.

Camille Nebeker, Ed.D., M.S., is an associate professor of behavioral medicine in the Department of Family Medicine and Public Health in the School of Medicine at the University of California, San Diego. Her research and teaching focus on two intersecting areas, community research capacity building (e.g., citizen science and community engaged research) and digital health research ethics (e.g., consent, privacy expectations, data management). She co-founded and directs the Research Center for Optimal Digital Ethics and leads the Building Research Integrity and Capacity programs and the Connected and Open Research Ethics initiative. Dr. Nebeker's research has received continuous support from government, foundation, and industry sources since 2002.

Dan O'Connor, Ph.D., is the head of humanities and social science at Wellcome Trust. Wellcome Trust is an independent global charitable foundation dedicated to improving health by helping great ideas to thrive. In his role at Wellcome Trust, Dr. O'Connor directs Europe's largest bioethics research funding portfolio as well as overseeing all of Wellcome Trust's research outside of the biomedical sciences. He has a Ph.D. in the history of medicine and was previously on the faculty at the Johns Hopkins Berman Institute of Bioethics.

Pilar Ossorio, Ph.D., J.D., is a professor of law and bioethics at the University of Wisconsin–Madison (UW) and the ethics scholar-in-residence and program lead for the ethics program at the UW-affiliated Morgridge Institute for Research. She leads the research ethics consultation service for UW and has participated in numerous federal advisory committees and National Academies of Sciences, Engineering, and Medicine committees.

Dorothy Roberts, J.D., is the 14th Penn Integrates Knowledge Professor and the George A. Weiss University Professor of Law and Sociology at the University of Pennsylvania, with joint appointments in the departments of Africana studies and sociology and the law school, where she is the inaugural

Raymond Pace and Sadie Tanner Mossell Alexander Professor of Civil Rights. She is also the founding director of the Penn Program on Race, Science, and Society. An internationally recognized scholar, public intellectual, and social justice advocate, Ms. Roberts has written and lectured extensively on the interplay of race and gender in U.S. institutions and has been a leader in transforming thinking on reproductive health, child welfare, and bioethics. She is the author of *Killing the Black Body: Race, Reproduction, and the Meaning of Liberty* (1997), *Shattered Bonds: The Color of Child Welfare* (2001), *Fatal Invention: How Science, Politics, and Big Business Re-create Race in the Twenty-First Century* (2011), and more than 100 articles and book chapters as well as the co-editor of 6 books. She has served on the boards of directors of the American Academy of Political and Social Science, the Black Women's Health Imperative, and the National Coalition for Child Protection Reform, and her work has been supported by the American Council of Learned Societies, the National Science Foundation, the Robert Wood Johnson Foundation, the Harvard Program on Ethics and the Professions, and the Stanford Center for the Comparative Studies in Race and Ethnicity. Recent recognitions of her work include the Society of Family Planning 2016 Lifetime Achievement Award and American Psychiatric Association 2015 Solomon Carter Fuller Award. In 2017 she was elected to the National Academy of Medicine.

Carla Saenz, Ph.D., is the regional bioethics advisor at the Pan American Health Organization (PAHO), which is the World Health Organization's regional office for the Americas. She is responsible for PAHO's regional program on bioethics, which provides supports on bioethics to countries in Latin America and the Caribbean (e.g., strengthening national research ethics systems, integrating ethics in health-related work, and advancing capacity on bioethics). Dr. Saenz also manages PAHO's ethics review committee, which reviews research conducted with PAHO's involvement in the region. An elected fellow of The Hastings Center, she has authored numerous publications on different areas of bioethics, co-edited the book *Public Health Ethics: Cases Spanning the Globe*, and contributed to several ethics guidance documents. She has been responsible for the development of PAHO's Zika virus ethics guidance. She holds a Ph.D. in philosophy from The University of Texas at Austin, and before joining PAHO she was at the Department of Bioethics at the Clinical Center of the National Institutes of Health and on the faculty of the Philosophy Department at the University of North Carolina at Chapel Hill.

Suchi Saria, Ph.D., is the John C. Malone Assistant Professor of Computer Science at the Johns Hopkins University Whiting School of Engineering, a professor of health system informatics at the School of Medicine, and a professor of health policy and management at the Bloomberg School of Public Health. She is the director of the Machine Learning, Artificial Intelligence, and Healthcare Lab and the founding research director of the Malone Center for Engineering in Healthcare at Johns Hopkins University. Her research has pioneered the development of next-generation diagnostic and treatment planning tools that use statistical machine learning methods to individualize care. In dealing with sepsis, a life-threatening condition, her work first demonstrated the use of machine learning to integrate diverse signals to make early detection possible. In Parkinson's disease, her work showed a first demonstration of using readily available sensors to easily track and measure symptom severity at home, which can serve to optimize treatment management. Her work has received recognition in numerous forms, including selection by IEEE Intelligent Systems to Artificial Intelligence's "10 to Watch" (2015), the DARPA Young Faculty Award (2016), *MIT Technology Review*'s "35 Innovators under 35" (2017), the prestigious Sloan Research Fellowship (2018), and the World Economic Forum Young Global Leader (2018). In 2017 her work was among four research contributions presented by Dr. France Córdova, the director of the National Science Foundation, to the House Commerce, Justice, Science, and Related Agencies Appropriations Committee. She was invited to join the National Academy of Engineering's Frontiers of Engineering in 2017 and to the National Academy of Medicine's Emerging Leaders in Health and Medicine. Dr. Saria received her undergraduate degree from Mount Holyoke College. She earned her M.Sc. and Ph.D. from Stanford University working with Dr. Daphne Koller. She visited Harvard University for a year as a National Science Foundation Computing Innovation fellow. Dr. Saria joined the Johns Hopkins faculty in 2012.

Tania Simoncelli, M.S., has designed advocacy strategies and policy solutions to address complex issues at the intersection of science, technology, law, and ethics for the past 20 years. In 2017 she joined the Chan Zuckerberg Initiative as the director of science policy, where her work focuses on enhancing public trust in and support for science and building an initiative to promote patient-driven disease research at scale. Prior to this, Ms. Simoncelli worked for the Broad Institute of the Massachusetts Institute of Technology and Harvard University as a senior advisor to Eric Lander and the executive director of Count Me In, an initiative that aims to accelerate biomedical research by facilitating patient–researcher partnerships. From 2010 to 2015 Ms. Simoncelli served in senior staff roles in the Obama administration, including as assistant director for forensic science and biomedical innovation within the White House Office of Science and Technology Policy, where she crafted a series of interagency forensic science reform efforts and helped drive the creation and launch of the President's Precision Medicine Initiative. From 2003 to 2010, Ms. Simoncelli worked for the American Civil Liberties Union as the organization's first-ever science advisor, where she spearheaded the organization's successful Supreme Court case challenging the patenting of human genes. In 2013 Ms. Simoncelli was named by the journal *Nature* as one of "10 people who mattered this year" for her work in ending gene patenting. She holds a B.A. in biology and society from Cornell University and an M.S. in energy and resources from the University of California, Berkeley, and she is the co-author with Sheldon Krimsky of *Genetic Justice: DNA Data Banks, Criminal Investigations, and Civil Liberties.*

Michael Summers, Ph.D., earned his B.S. in chemistry from the University of West Florida in 1980 and received his Ph.D. in 1984 in bioinorganic chemistry from Emory University. His laboratory has worked in the area of biological magnetic resonance spectroscopy for nearly 30 years. Dr. Summers has served terms on two National Institutes of Health (NIH) study sections and has been continuously funded by NIH since 1989 (including 20 years of NIH MERIT support). He has also been a Howard Hughes Medical Institute (HHMI) investigator for more than 20 years and was elected to the National Academy of Sciences in 2016. Dr. Summers and his team recently developed a novel nuclear magnetic resonance (NMR) method that enabled structural probing of the intact HIV-1 5′-leader (>700 nucleotide dimer) and showed that the leader undergoes dimerization-dependent remodeling; they also determined the NMR structure of a minimal region of the HIV-1 leader sufficient to direct RNA packaging. He has mentored 47 graduate students (66 percent women) and 24 postdoctoral fellows (58 percent women). Examples of female postdocs who successfully matriculated to research-intensive faculty positions include Victoria D'Souza (full professor with tenure at Harvard), Sepideh Khorasanizadeh (rose to full professor at the University of Virginia, now at the Burnham Institute), and Xiao Heng (tenure-track assistant professor at the University of Missouri–Columbia). Dr. Summers also directs an HHMI education grant program at the University of Maryland, Baltimore County, that supports high-achieving underrepresented-minority (URM) undergraduates and an NIH Initiative for Maximizing Student Development–supported program for diversifying graduate programs, which now supports more than 80 URM Ph.D. students. For his mentoring activities he has received the Ruth Kirschstein Award of the American Society for Biochemistry and Molecular Biology (2014), the Carl Bränden Award of the Protein Society (2011), the American Association for the Advancement of Science Mentor Award (2003), the Emily M. Gray Award for Biophysical Society (2003), and the White House Presidential Award for Science Mentoring (2000).

John Wilbanks is the chief commons officer at Sage Bionetworks. Previously Mr. Wilbanks worked as a legislative aide to Congressman Fortney "Pete" Stark, served as the first assistant director at Harvard's Berkman Center for Internet and Society, founded and led to acquisition the bioinformatics company Incellico, Inc., and was the executive director of the Science Commons project at Creative Commons. In February 2013, in response to a We the People petition that was spearheaded by Mr. Wilbanks and signed by 65,000 people, the U.S. government announced a plan to open up taxpayer-funded research data and make it available for free. Mr. Wilbanks holds a B.A. in philosophy from Tulane University and also studied modern letters at the Sorbonne.

Benjamin S. Wilfond, M.D., is the director of the Treuman Katz Center for Pediatric Bioethics and a pulmonologist at Seattle Children's Hospital. He is a professor and the chief of the Division of Bioethics and Palliative Care in the Department of Pediatrics at the University of Washington School of Medicine. He conducts empirical research and conceptual scholarship focused on ethical and policy issues at the research–clinical care interface. His current focus relates to the integration of genomic testing into clinical practice, informed consent about research on medical practices, and decision making about technological interventions in children with disabilities. He is the research ethics case co-editor of the *American Journal of Bioethics* and on the editorial boards of *The Hastings Center Report*, *Ethics and Human Research*, and the *Journal of Genetic Counseling*. He is a member of the U.S. Food and Drug Administration's Pediatrics Advisory Committee and the Standing Committee on Ethics at the Canadian Institutes of Health Research. He is a past president of the Association of Bioethics Program Directors and has served on the American Academy of Pediatrics Committee on Bioethics, the American Society of Human Genetics Social Issues Committee, and the American Thoracic Society Bioethics Taskforce. He is an elected member of the American Pediatric Society and a fellow of The Hastings Center. He attended Muhlenberg College and the New Jersey Medical School and completed his postgraduate training at the University of Wisconsin. He has held faculty appointments at the University of Arizona, the National Institutes of Health, and Johns Hopkins University. He is the founder and the former chair of the National Human Genome Research Institute intramural institutional review board (IRB) and has 30 years of experience on IRBs and data-monitoring committees and as a bioethics consultant.

Appendix C

Statement of Task

A planning committee of the National Academies of Sciences, Engineering, and Medicine will be appointed to conduct a 1-day workshop to bring together stakeholders to discuss potential ethical issues that may arise from new and emerging trends in biomedical research (including behavioral and social research) and society. The workshop will identify a range of current and emerging bioethical issues—both in basic and in clinical research—and explore a broad range of stakeholder perspectives. Input will be sought from a variety of perspectives, which may include patients/participants/individuals, bioethicists, academic and industry researchers, clinicians, and government representatives. The workshop will describe the state of the emerging science and potential pressing, recurring, emerging, and/or anticipated future bioethical issues in biomedical research and society that fall within the scope of the research and policy activities of the National Institutes of Health. Potential topics may include

- Use of digital technologies, artificial intelligence, and machine learning in biomedical research and clinical care;
- Emerging ethical challenges for sharing data from human research participants and use of human biospecimens;
- Health equity and health disparities in research, including
  - Recognizing and addressing barriers to participation in research and clinical care across diverse populations and groups,
  - Understanding the impact of cultural and social context on health and disease, and
  - Equitable distribution of the benefits and burdens of research;

- Innovative study designs, including crowdsourcing of research and citizen science;
- Novel approaches for enhancing bioethics infrastructure and training;
- New means for assessing and enhancing scientific workforce diversity; and/or
- Innovative solutions for enhancing research oversight infrastructure.

Given the broad scope of bioethical issues in research and the difficulty in addressing all possible issues in a single workshop, the following topics fall outside the scope of this workshop as they are being addressed in multiple other venues: gene editing, gene drives, human–animal chimera research, human fetal tissue research, neuroethics, and animal care and welfare. The planning committee will develop the agenda for the workshop, select and invite speakers and discussants, and moderate or identify moderators for the discussions. A workshop proceedings will be prepared by a designated rapporteur based on the information gathered and discussions held during the workshop in accordance with National Academies institutional policies and procedures.

Appendix D

Registered Attendees

Diaa Ahmed
American Association for the
    Advancement of Science

Seun Ajiboye
American Association for Dental
    Research

Adriana Bankston
Office of Federal Governmental
    Relations
University of California

Jeannie Baumann
Bloomberg Law

Inna Belfer
National Center for
    Complementary and
    Integrative Health
National Institutes of Health

Adam Berger
National Institutes of Health

Karen Bienstock
National Institutes of Health

Katherine D. Blizinsky
National Institutes of Health

Juliana Blome
Tribal Health Research Office
National Institutes of Health

Lawrence Brody
National Human Genome Research
    Institute

Jonca Bull
Strategic Regulatory Consultants

Charlisse Caga-anan
National Cancer Institute
National Institutes of Health

Alexander Capron
University of Southern California

Subhashini Chandresekharan
All of Us
National Institutes of Health

Karla Childers
Johnson & Johnson

Alicia Chou
National Institutes of Health

Caroline Cilio
Genentech

Elaine Collier
National Institutes of Health

Katharine Cooper
National Institutes of Health

David Curry
GE2P2 Global Foundation

Liza Dawson
Walter Reed Army Institute of
    Research

Megan Doerr
Sage Bionetworks

Gerald Dryden
University of Louisville

Helena Duncan
College of American Pathologists

Christen Elledge
Johns Hopkins University School
    of Medicine

Glenn Ellis
Strategies for Well-being, LLC

Nancy Emenaker
National Cancer Institute
National Institutes of Health

Katelyn Esmonde
Johns Hopkins Berman Institute of
    Bioethics

Rachel Fabi
SUNY Upstate Medical University

Shari Feirman
National Institutes of Health

Shannon Firth
MedPage Today

Grace Fisher-Adams
California Institute of Technology

Jason Gerson
Patient-Centered Outcomes
    Research Institute

Tina Getachew
American College of Radiology

Elena Ghanaim
National Human Genome
    Research Institute
National Institutes of Health

Melissa Goldstein
The George Washington University

Pamela González
Edudown Chile

Christine Grady
National Institutes of Health
    Clinical Center

Daria Grayer
Association of American Medical
   Colleges

Marielle Gross
Johns Hopkins Berman Institute of
   Bioethics

Chris Gunter
National Institutes of Health

Ilana Harrus
American Association for the
   Advancement of Science

Jaime Hernandez
Office of the Assistant Secretary
   for Health
U.S. Department of Health and
   Human Services

Tina Hernandez-Boussard
Stanford University

Gonzalo Hormazabel
Clinica Alemana Temuco

Kathy Hudson
Hudson Works LLC

Carol Hullin
Center of Digital Innovation

Shanda Hunt
Office of the President
University of California

Luz Huntington Moskos
University of Louisville

Audrey Jackson
American Association for Cancer
   Research

Praduman Jain
Vibrent Health

Mariel Jais
The George Washington University

Liza Johnson
St. Jude Children's Research
   Hospital

Lyric Jorgensen
National Institutes of Health

Julie Kaneshiro
Office for Human Research
   Protections
U.S. Department of Health and
   Human Services

Dave Kaufman
National Human Genome
   Research Institute
National Institutes of Health

Naomi Kawin

Sallie Keller
University of Virginia

Dave Klein
Vibrent Health

Barbara Koenig
University of California, San
   Francisco

Naoru Koizumi
George Mason University

Catharine Krebs
Physicians Committee for
   Responsible Medicine

Carleigh Krubiner
Center for Global Development

Cathryn Lee
U.S. Food and Drug Administration

Chengyuan Li
National Institutes of Health

Nicole Lockhart
National Human Genome
    Research Institute
National Institutes of Health

Yuan Luo
National Institutes of Health

Mario Macis
Johns Hopkins University

Maria Madison
Brandeis University

Punam Mathur
National Institute of Allergy and
    Infectious Diseases
National Institutes of Health

Molly McGinnis
American Society of Clinical
    Oncology

Jerry Menikoff
Office of the Assistant Secretary
    for Health
U.S. Department of Health and
    Human Services

Nancy Miller
National Cancer Institute
National Institutes of Health

Wilhelmine Miller

Helen Moore
National Cancer Institute
National Institutes of Health

Rhonda Moore
U.S. Food and Drug Administration

Karen Near
U.S. Agency for International
    Development

Michael Nestor
U.S. Department of Energy

Carmelle Norice-Ta
National Institutes of Health

Gary Norman
Centers for Medicare & Medicaid
    Services

Joyce Nortey
Evidation Health

Miriam O'Day
Alpha-1 Foundation

Laura Odwazny
U.S. Department of Health and
    Human Services

Pilar Ossorio
University of Wisconsin

Vivian Ota Wang
National Cancer Institute
National Institutes of Health

Taunton Paine
Office of Science Policy
National Institutes of Health

Diana Pankevich
Pfizer Inc.

George Papanicolaou
National Heart, Lung, and Blood
    Institute
National Institutes of Health

Jennifer Plank-Bazinet
National Institutes of Health

Ivor Pritchard
Office of the Assistant Secretary
    for Health
U.S. Department of Health and
    Human Services

Chelsea Ratcliff
University of Utah

Barbara Redman
New York University

Gabriela Riscuta
National Cancer Institute
National Institutes of Health

Carol Robertson-Plouch
Convergence Bioscience LLC

Deborah Runkle
American Association for the
    Advancement of Science

Maya Sabatello
Columbia University

Christy Sandborg
Stanford University

Victor Schneider
Office of the Chief Health and
    Medical Officer
NASA

Yalini Senathirajah
University of Pittsburgh Medical
    School

Stephanie Shipp
Social and Decision Analytics
University of Virginia

Jeffrey Sich
The George Washington University

Kevin A. Smith
Roper St. Francis Healthcare

Robert A. Sorenson
National Institute of Allergy and
    Infectious Diseases
National Institutes of Health

Scott Steele
University of Rochester

Nidhi Subbaraman
Nature

Joanna Szczepanik
National Institute of Mental
    Health
National Institutes of Health

Jim Taylor
National Institutes of Health

Ericka Thomas
All of Us
National Institutes of Health

Darla Thompson
American Association for the
    Advancement of Science

Alyssa Tonsing-Carter
National Institutes of Health

Michelle Tregear
National Breast Cancer Coalition

Ellen Wann
National Institutes of Health

Jithesh Weetil
Medical Device Innovation
    Consortium

Leah White
American Society of Addiction
    Medicine

Cheri Wiggs
National Eye Institute

David Wilson
National Institutes of Health

Gerald Winslow
Loma Linda University